MW00636947

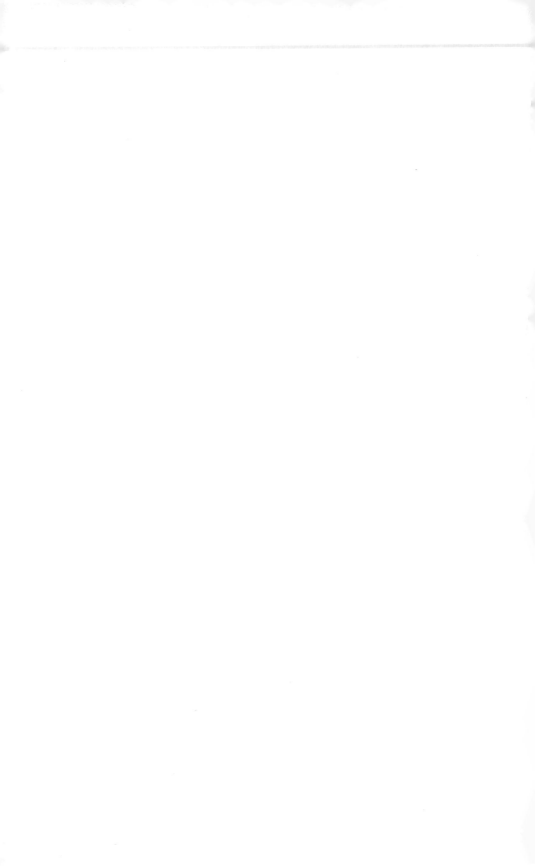

SUCKERED

The History Of Sugar

Our Toxic Addiction

Our Power to Change

JEFFREY EISENBERG, M.D.

WITH SANDRA CANOSA

Lawless Publishing, LLC

| Florida |

Lawless Publishing, LLC
530 Ocean Drive #501
Juno Beach, FL 33408

First edition: September 2015
Designer: Connor Smith
Set in Minion Pro

ISBN 978-0-9967-1160-9

Printed by Mercury Print Productions, Inc., 2015 in the Unites States of America

This book is dedicated to
the two-thirds of Americans who are overweight or obese,
the one-half that are pre-diabetic or overtly diabetic,
the one-third who are hypertensive,
and those of us who unknowingly are next to join these ranks.

CONTENTS

Part IV. Sugarholics:
Your Brain on Sugar

Part V. Public Policy:
Dealing With Sugar

Part VI. Epilogue

Introduction

True Confessions

"**H**ello…MY NAME IS JEFF AND I'M A SUGAR ADDICT." If there were a Sugarholics Anonymous group, that would be my introduction. The group would respond, "Hi Jeff" and I would recount my story:

I have been a sugar addict for as long as I can remember. As a child, I was often rewarded with candy — Raisinettes were my favorite. The ice cream man was a superhero in my neighborhood. When his truck bells rang, I salivated like a Pavlovian dog. If I had a nightmare, my dad would offer me a cinnamon bun to settle me down. Pop-Tarts were a vitamin-infused staple in our house. I was convinced we had a chocolate cow. Advertising during Saturday morning cartoons only reinforced my behavior. Like every other kid, I was "cuckoo for Cocoa Puffs"!

Fast-forward to adulthood. At restaurants, I always looked at the dessert menu first — dinner was just in the way. I had secret stashes of dark chocolate, and the sight of a Klondike bar made those ice-cream-truck bells go off in my head. My conference table at work always had a smorgasbord of donuts, cakes and cookies. I was drinking two "energy drinks" a day. Sugar was interwoven into every facet of my daily routine.

But I was in shape! I have always been a compulsive exerciser. I played multiple sports in high school and ran long distances in college. I took up biking in my forties and was a cult follower of P-90X and Insanity. I was never overweight. And my main meals were quite healthy.

So imagine my indignation when, at age 45, my physician informed me I had high blood pressure, a very low "protective" cholesterol (HDL), and a fasting glucose that was creeping out of the normal range. I was incredulous! I cursed my family history. And I cursed the blood pressure pills he prescribed me.

A few years later, I started to experience occasional joint discomfort. At times, I couldn't wear my wedding and college rings because my fingers were swollen and stiff. I was frequently drained of energy. I would nap like a puppy.

Sadly, I realized I wasn't alone. You see, the Sugarholics Anonymous groups are standing-room-only.

I have been practicing in private Pediatrics for nearly three decades. I have witnessed extraordinary medical advances: Babies born three months premature can now thrive, and a child with Leukemia (ALL) has a greater than 85% chance for full recovery. But there's also a cultural and societal epidemic raging.

Take J.P., a 17-year-old patient who transferred into my practice. His mother had gestational diabetes during pregnancy, and he was nine pounds at birth. He was fed infant formula until a year of age, at which point he was the average size of a 22-month-old. He had been introduced to organic jars of baby food, all-natural juices, and a mixed variety of baby yogurt. The cereals he ate all boasted "carefully selected whole grain oats." All this was quite normal. But over the ensuing years, his meal portions grew larger and he became progressively more sedentary. (As you will see in this book, this "overconsumption" phenomenon was not a choice as much as a biochemical outcome).

J.P., a teenager, now weighs 288 pounds and is fighting an uphill metabolic battle. And his case isn't unusual. One out of four children now in my practice are considered obese. And 1/3 of the newly diagnosed type 2 diabetics today are children. I see a worrisome increase in the incidence of lipid abnormalities and associated hypertension. And all of this is occurring while doctors are stressing healthy eating habits and the benefits of exercise.

It doesn't stop there. Currently 2/3 of adults are overweight or obese, 1/2 are pre-diabetic (many without realizing it) or overtly diabetic, and 1/3 have hypertension. Last year we spent 445 billion of our health care dollars trying to treat these diseases. Only the pharmaceutical companies are thriving.

So what's behind this disaster? That's what this book will explain, along with the best way to fix the problem — both on a large scale, and individually for each of us. With a look at history, science, the latest research, and politics, we'll show a hard-to-swallow truth: Refined sugar has emerged as the new silent killer in our society.

We'll start with the strangely fascinating history of sugar — how it became a priceless commodity for royalty, how wars were fought over it, how it changed the lives of famous people from Napoleon to Gandhi. And all the while, we'll show how it was undermining whole cultures and health.

As we reach more modern history, we'll cover some shocking truths about sugar in this country, including devious advertising practices and lobbying that helped create a near-universal sugar addiction in our culture. And then we'll show how, in the early '70s, a tragic mistake was made: Instead of focusing on the evidence that sugar was ruining our health, nutritionists (and the government) made fat the enemy. And what happened? Fat consumption decreased, yet the incidence of coronary heart disease, obesity, and diabetes dramatically increased.

The science we present will show why this mistake was so costly — both in actual expense to society, and in human lives lost and affected. Trust me, when you read the research in this book (even if you didn't like science classes in school), I believe you'll be shocked and convinced that we need to make a big change.

It seems impossible that sweet, innocent refined sugar can be so deadly. It's why the food industry was able to add even more sugar to foods to replace the decrease in fat, which has made things that much worse. Today, 80% of the items in grocery stores have added sugar. But by the time you finish this book, I'm convinced you'll understand what I came to realize: Sugar is toxic, and it's at the heart of this terrible, self-induced health epidemic we're facing.

You see, for me it's professional *and* personal. That patient I mentioned, J.P.? Really the only difference between him and me was the additional weight he held. Metabolically, we were both a mess. (As it turns out, as many as 40% of normal-weight individuals are in metabolic disarray, while 20% of obese individuals have normal metabolic profiles). Excess sugar was the pitfall he and I shared.

When I realized medication wasn't helping me, I began to research what chronic added sugar can do to a person's health. Remarkably, there are generations of books and articles citing the adverse effects of sugar; most of us (me included) just haven't been reading.

So I became a "born again" eater. I cut my intake of added sugar to less than 25 grams a day. It wasn't easy, especially because the reward center of our brains is wired to keep us eating sweet stuff. But I became Sherlock Holmes, finding the hidden sugar that's in virtually every packaged food out there. It was me against the food industry—the evil empire sugar-coating our food with reckless abandon.

I shunned man-made, processed food in favor of more fiber, protein and, yes, healthy fat. I drank only water. And eventually, the cravings grew less intense.

One month in, I noticed a dramatic metamorphosis. I had more energy. I no longer needed to nap. My exercise routines were more efficient. My mood improved. And, I stopped taking my blood pressure medicine! I could put my rings back on. My "protective cholesterol" increased 33%. I noticed that my acid reflux symptoms all but abated, and I was able to stop my antacids for the first time in over a decade!

I began to share my experience with patients. The parents of my patients became interested, too, and asked for guidance. I studied my patients' lab results before and after reducing sugar consumption. Not surprisingly, their labs also began to normalize, and their testimonials were overwhelmingly positive.

You might feel pretty healthy now, but from experiences in my medical practice and in my own life, I know that feeling can be deceiving. And I know what's at stake, for our society and for each and every one of us. This book is the first step on a journey of awareness and redemption that will lead to a healthier, longer, and more productive life.

   –Jeffrey Eisenberg, M.D.

PART I:

WHITE GOLD

The Root of the Problem

CHAPTER 1

Raising Cane

Ancient History

Hurts So Good

SUGAR IS A PROBLEM 10,000 years in the making. It's not something we think about as we bite into a candy bar, but whole kingdoms triumphed from sugar. Countries invaded because of it. Prominent figures such as Christopher Columbus, Napoleon, and Fidel Castro changed history with it. And millions have died from being forced to cultivate it.

Understanding the extent to which sugar came to dominate world affairs can help us see how it has come to saturate our own current diet. Ironically, the real problem stems from the fact that sugar — in its natural form, sugarcane — is a practically perfect food.

Ounce for ounce, sugarcane is one of the most calorie-dense foods on the planet in its raw state. And at the dawn of the agricultural age, humans had to work hard to get calories.

Some 10,000 years ago or so, the inhabitants of the island of New Guinea developed a way to dig shallow wells in the rich soil to grow taro, bananas, yams, and sugarcane. Sugarcane in particular became an important part of the ancient Oceania diet. It nourished bodies and filled bellies. Two-thirds of the plant is made up of water; the remaining third is half fiber, half sucrose. When chewed raw, cane comes packed with proteins, B vitamins, potassium, iron, calcium, and sodium.

Of course, ancient civilizations had no idea about all that. They just knew the taste was delicious, and chewing the cane gave them energy. New Guinea was relatively isolated in the Pacific, but its agricultural ideas and crops slowly spread, reaching as far as Hawaii and the Indian subcontinent. Sugarcane became one of the most impressive and lucrative foods for farming. An ancient Polynesian creation myth has it that the first woman emerged from a stalk of sugarcane, and from her was birthed all of mankind. In India, too, sugarcane became incredibly important. It was used as an offering in religious ceremonies, fed to cows as a sacred crop, and administered liberally to the sick for its supposed medicinal or even magical properties.[1]

Clearly there was something in this plant that other plants lacked — something that made it so perfectly sweet. Perhaps as early as 800 BCE, Indians developed a method to squeeze the juices out of a sugarcane reed using a mechanical press. They then boiled the juices until all water had evaporated and only chunks of crystallized sucrose — pure sugar — remained. Depending on the quality and purity of the crystals, sugar was called *khaṇda* or *śarkarā* in ancient Sanskrit—the basis for the English words *candy* and *sugar.*[2]

But that process of separating the sugar also strips away the protective fiber and removes those essential vitamins and minerals. In later chapters, we'll see how such refined sugar wreaks havoc in our bodies. For now, suffice it to say that sugar has been damaging us for many centuries.

Sugar School

What's remarkable is that the unhealthy effects of sugar have been known for many centuries.

By around 300 BCE, the technologies for refining and producing sugar had spread from India throughout the Mid-East, becoming increasingly sophisticated and efficient as the centuries wore on. But even by the 5th century CE, pure sugar was still too expensive and scarce to be used every day, even by the wealthy. On holidays, Persian kings celebrated with a breakfast of "white sugar with fresh Indian nuts."[3] Weddings and celebrations became a kind of competitive show: families would commission fantastic, over-the-top, and obscenely expensive sculptures made from marzipan — a blend of sugar and almond paste — simply to display their extravagant wealth.

The Persian Empire was, at the time, one of the wealthiest and most innovative cultures in the world. It established one of the world's first formal schools, the Academy of Gondishapur, in what is now western Iran. Gondishapur was an educational and research institution, with scientists, engineers, and doctors working side-by-side to improve production methods of sugar as well as establish new medical and commercial uses for it. New extraction and refining techniques were developed, and the sugar itself was widely prescribed as an elixir for treating kidney and bladder problems as well as asthma and respiratory afflictions.

At the same time, the consequences of overindulging in sugar had become apparent. Too much sugar was noted to cause tooth decay, excess liver bile, and — in extreme and prolonged cases — the unusual passage of sugars through urine. A sickly sweet smell to the urine — a symptom we now recognize as the calling card of diabetes — was, at the time, a death sentence.

Those doctors even recognized a difference between types of diabetes that developed suddenly in childhood and the kind that developed later in life as a result of eating too much sugar (what we now distinguish as Type 1 and Type 2 diabetes). Even so, the mechanisms behind the disease were poorly understood and untreatable. It almost always resulted in a slow and painful demise for the patient.

Even as Gondishapur was discovering the ill effects of sugar, its academics were also developing ways to make crystallized sugar ever more pure and refined. When all of the moisture content from the sugarcane's water is removed, sugar can last, unspoiled, for a very long time. Its stability, combined with its high caloric content, made sugar an invaluable food resource for armies on the move. Ironically, it was sugar that helped fuel the Muslim armies that eventually conquered the Persian Empire by the year 651.

Sweet Routes

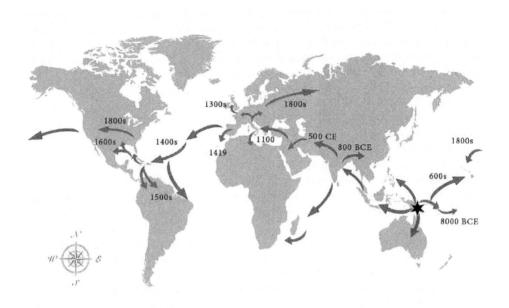

Sugar's relentless spread across the globe continued. Between the years 1095 and 1291, the Crusades that pitted Christians against Muslims led to the creation of extensive routes across Europe to transport men and goods from the north to the battlegrounds of the Mid-East. As soldiers and suppliers returned, they brought with them crafts, goods, and foods — especially sugar, tea, and spices — never before seen in Europe. Even as the Crusades proved a losing battle for the Christians, trade between the two cultures continued to flourish. The Italian port cities of Genoa, Venice, and Pisa proved especially influential in establishing routes of international trade long after the wars had ended.

Still, it took time and expense to transport goods such as sugar from so far away. The first written mention of sugar in the English language doesn't appear until around 1300, from an account in London, England. At the time, a single teaspoon of white sugar crystals cost the modern-day equivalent of five dollars, making a sweetened cup of tea a lavish affair indeed.[4] To put this into perspective, using this price conversion, a 12 oz. can of Coca Cola containing

39 g of sugar would have cost nearly $49 just for the sugar alone, and for a 20 oz. bottle the sugar cost would be $81.

Sugar at the time was considered a spice, much like other popular Eastern imports such as peppercorn, ginger, and cinnamon. But unlike those spices, sugar could be used in much greater quantities to an even greater effect. Too much cinnamon might cause you to gag, but there seemed to be no limit to how much sugar the tongue could enjoy. Entire meals in the royal courts of Europe were sometimes made solely from sugar.

As sugar remained expensive, it was a great status symbol in medieval Europe, just as it was in the old Persia. The more sugar a host could bestow upon and display to his guests, the more affluent and generous he appeared. The courts of England, France, Spain, and Portugal often tried to out-sweet each other, from ornate sugar-sculpture decorations to plates and bowls made out of sugar paste. Even the after-dinner playing cards could be shaped from hardened and painted sheets of sugar.

Cheap Labor and the New World

As the demand for sugar in Europe grew, eager businessmen sought to bring sugarcane closer to Europe. And sugar's ill effects began to spread to these societies as well.

Cane farms were cultivated on the islands of Cyprus and Sicily, giving the Italian port cities greater control over their sugar product. But the Mediterranean climate was not hot and humid enough to grow cane well, and European refining methods weren't as sophisticated as those in the Middle East. So the Europeans could only compete by keeping prices lower than their rivals', which they did by forcing indigenous island peasants or prisoners from nearby lands to work the cane fields under feudal, slave-like conditions.

Demand grew no matter how much growers produced or importers traded. The small islands of the Mediterranean were maxed out with sugarcane by the 1400s. But soon, a fluke would usher in a new era of sugar production — and of human exploitation.

In 1419, a couple of Portuguese ships were blown off course on their way to Africa. They landed on a densely wooded, subtropical island completely uninhabited by humans. They promptly claimed it for the Kingdom of Portugal and named it Madeira, the Portuguese word for "wood."

The rich, wooded land of Madeira created a profitable lumber industry for western Europe, and as forest and trees were cleared, new crops were planted in their place. The hot and humid setting proved ideal for Portugal to produce one of Europe's best-loved crops: sugarcane.

Before the close of the 15th century, Madeira's sugar output was substantial enough to compete with Mediterranean production. Portugal modeled its business after its southern counterparts, employing convicts and debtors to work as indentured servants in the fields. When that labor force was exhausted, plantation owners turned to Africa, where they could exchange goods for more prisoners condemned to work the rest of their lives under cane.

The flood of new supplies of sugar on the European market drove prices down dramatically: In England, for example, the retail price of a pound of sugar went from 17 pence in 1470 to only four pence per pound, over a 76% decrease in price by 1500.[5] Thanks to the sugar business — and cheap labor — Portugal became a domineering financial and political force over all of Europe.

Next door to Portugal, the newly united Kingdom of Spain was eager to secure a similar foothold in global affairs. So it financed an Italian explorer named Christopher Columbus, who sought a westward water passage to India. That 1492 voyage, of course, actually brought him to parts of what are now the Bahamas, Cuba, and Hispaniola (the island that today is split between the Dominican Republic and Haiti). But Columbus thought he was in the Orient, where the potential was enormous. Columbus gained backing to return to what he thought was the "New World" fourteen months later, bringing with him the same crop that had revolutionized Portugal's economy on Madeira: sugarcane.

White Gold

After news of Columbus's journeys spread, various kingdoms quickly realized how much land still remained unseen or unclaimed. Any indigenous people, it seemed, could easily be conquered through western advantages such as firepower, horsepower, and disease.

The race for global territorial expansion — and riches — was on. Though the lure of gold enticed many explorers and *conquistadors*, the absence of precious metals in the new lands could easily be solved by planting a few acres of sugarcane, which was nearly as lucrative as gold itself. Colonists and consumers alike called refined sugar crystals "white gold."

Sugarcane was not native to any American lands, but it flourished in the equatorial regions of the Caribbean islands, Brazil, and the northeastern cape of South America. By the mid-1600s, sugarcane had become the dominant crop of the New World. Vast tracts of arable land made it possible for growers to expand cultivation and produce more sugar at cheaper prices than even the Middle East could.

Yet sugar remained primarily a status symbol for the wealthy, especially as kingdoms in Europe established their own private line of sugar colonies. Elizabeth I of England was said to be so fond of sugar that her dinners of sweetmeats were followed by candied fruits and sugar-laden wine. Elizabeth was also known among diplomats and associates for her rotted black teeth, late in her life.

The lands best suited for sugarcane emerged as the most profitable and coveted acquisitions among European powers. The British-controlled Barbados, for example, an island smaller in area than the city of Chicago, conducted more trade than any other English colony throughout the globe during the 17th century; 90% of that trade directly involved sugar.

In 1697, the French and the Spanish battled for control over the island of Hispaniola, considered the "Pearl of the Antilles" for its tremendous sugar output. Eventually, the western third of the island was ceded to the French, which they named Saint-Domingue, and the rest remained with the Spanish, called Santo Domingo. The political, cultural, and language barriers established then still remain as the independent nations of Haiti and the Dominican Republic.

The Portuguese remained a dominant force in overseas expansion with its claims to the massive area of Brazil, which throughout the colonial era and up to this day serves as the world's leading grower and refiner of sugars. Danish, Dutch, Prussian, and Swedish colonists also dominated various islands of the Caribbean; sometimes the same land would change hands multiple times between ruling countries. The lust for sugar was becoming a rush to conquer lands. And when a land was conquered, its people were ripe for exploitation.

How to Run a Sugar Plantation

Even to this day, the most successful sugarcane farms are large-scale, mono-crop productions. A producer's ability to manufacture and refine sugar is limited only by the amount of cane he can process in a refinery. Not surprisingly, it requires a lot of manpower to keep a sugar production up and running.

To man their fields and mills, European plantation owners first forced the indigenous people of the Caribbean and the Americas, usually taken as prisoners of war, into labor. And that labor was — and remains — grueling.

Workers have to tend to the cane as it grows, cut it down when it's ready, transport the heavy stalks from field to mill, process the cane through machines, extract the juice, strip the fiber, oversee the boiling of the juices, transport the juices from one vat to another for refinement, then package, ship, and sell the final product.

Each stalk of cane is a good three inches in diameter, and over six feet high. The thick, fibrous reeds must be chopped down by hand, one by one. The ground it grows in is typically wet, soggy, and uneven. Excess leaves on top — the "trash" — must be removed or they'll clog the refining machines. Harvest begins in June and lasts through the fall months, when temperatures in the Caribbean can approach 100 degrees and humidity is at its peak. Few people would ever willingly take up the work.

As production expanded — and as native populations were increasingly decimated by war and disease — landowners required additional workers. A triangle of barter developed: American goods including sugar and rum would be traded to Europe for fine goods, weapons, and textiles, which would be traded to Africa for slave laborers, which in turn would be traded back to the Americas for more sugar and rum.

Other crops and industries were of course involved in the African slave trade that crisscrossed the Atlantic Ocean for the next 300 years, but no business was as ruthless or dependent on forced human labor as the sugar industry. The plantations in particular produced some of the most brutal working conditions; the average life expectancy once a person was committed to slavery was only seven years.

Between Columbus' first step on American soil in 1492 and the last formal abolishment of slavery in the western hemisphere in 1888, an estimated ten million people were taken from Africa and sold into hard labor. Of those, four million were sold into slavery in Portuguese-controlled Brazil alone, where sugarcane rapidly took over the countryside.

A common 17th-century Portuguese saying said: "Without sugar, no Brazil; without slaves, no sugar; without Angola, no slaves."[6] Even as millions poured into the fields and countless more would be born into slavery every year, the death rate of slaves on many plantations exceeded the birth rate, and owners had to continuously replenish their working stock.

Sugar for the People

The expansion of the plantations plus cost benefits of economies of scale in sugar production gradually led to lower prices. Sugar, once a luxury for only the very rich, became increasingly affordable for the merchant classes, clergymen, and well-to-do housewives. Britain, with the key acquisition of the sugar island of Jamaica, began to surpass all other European countries in the race for colonization.

Public opinion about sugar was divided in 18th-century Britain. In 1715, a Dr. Frederick Slare published a widespread treatise called *A Vindication of*

Sugars, which advocated for the use of a pound of sugar every day, mixed in with food, drinks, wine, snuff, or even used as a hand lotion or tooth powder.

At the same time, Royal Court of England physician Thomas Willis blamed sugar for a host of new diseases crippling the country. Merchant sailors who transported sugar and rum across the ocean (and who ate a diet largely consisting of sugar and rum) were plagued with scurvy. Increasing tooth decay was noted among the wealthy. And, especially within the British royal court, a curious condition emerged where subjects emitted great amounts of sweet-smelling urine. Willis coined the ailment *diabetes mellitus*, from the Latin words "to siphon" and "sweet." The general public, however, typically just called it "the pissing evil."

As for the ruling class, the power of European nations increasingly resided in the wealth of their colonies. By the 1700s, England and France overtook Portugal and Spain as the world's largest producers of sugar; more than half of the world's entire product — more than 22,000 tons — came from French and British colonies in the Caribbean.[7]

With increased wealth, England and France also emerged as the dominant players in global affairs and international politics. More money from the profits of the sugar trade afforded them better armies, better palaces, and better political sway. But the very methods used to conquer the market — free trade, colonial favoritism, abuse of the land, and exploitative labor practices — would be the seeds of discontent that would eventually uproot the European colonial system itself.

CHAPTER 2

Liberté, Égalité, Sucre

Voices Against Slavery

"WHEN WE LABOR IN THE SUGAR WORKS, and the mill happens to snatch hold of a finger, they instantly chop off our hand; and when we attempt to run away, they cut off a leg. Both these cases have happened to me, and it is at this expense that you eat sugar in Europe." This story, told by a maimed slave in Voltaire's famous 1759 novel *Candide: Or, The Optimist*, ends with the lament, "Dogs, monkeys, and parrots are a thousand times less wretched than I." The character Candide can only burst into tears as he walks away.[8]

By the mid-18th century, it was clear to many that slavery was amoral. The Age of Enlightenment, with Voltaire as a leading voice, spoke of humanism, reasoning, and logic, and the ideas spread throughout Europe. Slavery and its connection with sugar was one of the movement's issues — an obvious example of the ills of the colonial system. Sugar quickly became the poster child of the abolitionist movement.

The Thirteen Colonies of North America were not immune. Even New England, though it didn't grow cane itself, was as entrenched in the sugar-slave relationship as any Caribbean colony. Harbors along Massachusetts and Rhode Island were major ports for receiving and selling off slaves brought in directly from African ships, and they also imported large shipments of raw molasses from the Caribbean to be made into rum.

The first commercial distillery in North America was founded in Boston in 1700. By 1770, there were at least 140 distilleries along the New England coast. Together, they produced more than five million gallons of rum derived from Caribbean sugar every year, which in turn was exported to the other side of the Atlantic or, as seemed more likely, drunk by the Colonialists themselves. Access to safe and clean drinking water was a problem in many Colonial settlements, so distilled rum often took its place at and between meals. Each Colonial American accounted for four gallons of rum consumed every year.[9]

Because much of the alcohol in America came from sugar itself, temperance movements, anti-sugar movements, and abolitionist movements often rallied together. The Anti-Saccharite Society of New England was a largely Quaker group that advocated for boycotts on slave-produced sugar and rum. An abolitionist pamphlet produced by the group reads: "Nay, so necessarily connected are our consumption of the commodity and the misery resulting from it, that in every pound of sugar used (the produce of slaves imported from Africa), we may be considered as consuming two ounces of human flesh... [One] cannot look on a piece of sugar without conceiving it stained with spots of human blood."[10]

But without the rum industry, the North American colonies had little else to stand on economically. Rum was Rhode Island's second-largest export throughout much of the 18th century, second only to candles.

A Bitter Tax

American rum producers, like much of the rest of the world, bought whatever sugar was cheapest on the market. In an effort to protect its colonial interests, England imposed a tax in 1733 on any sugar or molasses entering New England from non-British colonies. But the Molasses Act, as it was called, was routinely ignored. Next the crown imposed the Sugar Act of 1764, levying a heavy tax on any and all sugar in the North American colonies,

British or not. Royal soldiers were deployed to see that the tax was, this time, strictly enforced.

By this time, Colonial North America had one of the highest per capita sugar consumption rates in the world, second only to Britain.[11] The Sugar Act didn't just affect local rum producers and shipping companies; it manipulated the price of basic food costs for everyday citizens.

People were outraged by the new tax. Protests and riots, sometimes violent, ripped through New England's port cities. It was a matter of economics but also principle: colonists felt it was unfair to pass laws taxing the American people when they had no one to represent their voices or interests in Parliament. It was one of the first major tax acts that led to protests of "No taxation without representation," a decade before the better known Tea Act of 1773.

After Americans won independence from Great Britain, at the new nation's first inaugural ball, George Washington celebrated by serving his guests thirty gallons of the finest Barbados rum.

More Revolution

By the time America had gained independence from Great Britain, the French colony of Saint-Domingue — on the western side of the island of Hispaniola — was producing 40% of the world's sugar supply and 60% of its coffee, making it the single most valuable possession of the French Empire. Saint-Domingue was "the greatest colony in the world, the pride of France, and the envy of every other imperialist nation."[12]

France's portion of the island was inhabited by about 4,000 white colonists and some 500,000 black slaves. Conditions in the sugarcane and coffee fields of Saint-Domingue were reportedly some of the harshest in any of the Caribbean islands.

Two years after the French Revolution, on the night of August 22, 1791, thousands of slaves in Saint-Domingue rose up *en masse*. The revolt had been secretly organized by leaders once trained as warriors in Africa, but sold as captured prisoners to slave merchants and sent overseas. As the revolt spread, more and more slave groups joined in. The uprising succeeded: thousands of colonialists were killed, and 180 sugar plantations and hundreds more coffee farms were destroyed.

By the start of 1792, former slave revolutionaries controlled one-third of the colony. After another dozen years of struggle, all of the territory would belong to the rebels and be renamed: the Republic of Haiti.

Repercussions in the Homeland

The Haitian Revolution shocked the imperial sugar world. Many Europeans could not believe that black African slaves could possibly succeed against a nation of armed white colonists. More immediately, the global sugar market was thrown off balance. Supplies plummeted without Saint-Domingue's usual output and prices soared.

The loss was particularly acute in mainland France, and especially Paris, where urban food shortages were becoming increasingly problematic. The average Parisian consumed fifty pounds of sugar every year. In January of 1792, just as the events of Haiti climaxed, riots erupted along the streets of Paris. Five sugar storage houses were broken into, and two deliberately set on fire in protest of escalating food and sugar prices.

Civil unrest only continued and increased from then on, culminating in the arrest and later execution of King Louis XVI and his wife, Marie Antoinette. Marie's "Let them eat cake" quip had not been well received.

Vive le Sucre

By 1794, slavery in all French colonies, including Saint-Domingue, was formally abolished. Emancipation was a major victory for the Haitian rebels. But just five years later, Napoleon Bonaparte rose to power in France and, in 1802, re-instituted slavery in Saint-Domingue and the other French Caribbean colonies, hoping to revitalize the damaged sugar industry and also use the lands to gain better access to the underdeveloped French property in North America, the *Louisiane* territory.

A new surge of revolts erupted in Saint-Domingue, and Napoleon dispatched 30,000 troops to quash the rebellion once and for all. But in a true reversal of fortunes (centuries earlier, smallpox and other European-borne diseases infected and killed up to 95% of the pre-Columbian Native American population), over half of Napoleon's men caught yellow fever and died within the first two months of fighting in Saint-Domingue.

The Haitian rebels easily overpowered the rest of Napoleon's forces. Its ties with France severed, Haiti became the first independent nation of the Caribbean since before Columbus's arrival 312 years earlier.

Napoleon shifted his efforts to dominating mainland Europe. To pay for his wars, he sold off the entirety of the Louisiana Territory — 828,000 square miles of land stretching from New Orleans to Wyoming — to the United States for the incredible bargain of $15 million, or just four cents per acre.

The United States still relied on foreign imports for its sugar, unable to grow cane in its own climate. But the acquisition of Louisiana and the warm wetlands of the bayou allowed for domestic production. By 1860, the United States was producing nearly 300,000 tons of sugar every year — with the help of 300,000 slaves.[13]

Sugar Blockade

By the 19th century, sugar had become a staple of the European diet, especially as an accompaniment to coffee, tea, and sweetbreads. But still, consumption levels were nowhere near what they are today. The average annual consumption of sugar in Europe in 1800 was around eighteen pounds per person.[14] By comparison, most western European countries today consume well over 100 pounds per person per year, with Americans leading the charge at levels above 130 pounds per person.

Even with every inch of arable land in the New World planted with sugarcane, production at the beginning of the 19th century couldn't keep up with demand. So Napoleon turned to an old crop that held new potential: the beet.

Beets to the Rescue

In the 1760s, Prussian scientists had worked on developing a method to isolate the sucrose content of starchy root vegetables like beets and carrots. Their initial results were crude and inefficient, especially compared to sugarcane, and their research went largely unnoticed for decades.

Now, French scientists developed refinement methods that led to purified sucrose from white sugar beets that looked and tasted just like sugar from cane. In 1811, Napoleon dedicated over 65,000 acres of land to beet cultivation and donated one million francs to sugar beet research and production initiatives at schools and universities. The stimulus plan worked: by 1813, the amount of French soil planted with sugar beets had grown to 250,000 acres. These beets could go on to be processed into sugar at one of the country's 334 factory mills.[15]

The new technologies of sugar beet refining made it possible for other countries in temperate climate zones without a wealth of overseas colonies to start developing a sugar culture of their own. By the 1860s, refineries had been established in Belgium, the Netherlands, Poland, Sweden, and Russia. Before long, half of all sugar consumed in Europe was derived from beets instead of cane.[16]

Not coincidentally, the rise of beet sugar counteracted the decline of slavery in the western hemisphere. Beet production in Europe made the use of slave labor in far-off colonies appear increasingly unnecessary and inhumane. By the mid-19th century, nearly all European nations had renounced slavery or given up their colonial holdings in the Americas. Only Spain, the United States, and the newly independent nation of Brazil — all of whom relied on sugarcane as a vital cash crop — carried on with the institution of slavery.

The introduction of beet sugar flooded the market, and as prices fell, more consumers could buy more sugar. Between 1800 and 1900, the per capita consumption of sugar in most parts of Europe increased fivefold — from 18 pounds to 90 pounds per year.

The lust for sugar had reached the masses. And that meant the need for…even more sugar. War, slavery, revolution, disease: if any of this tainted the production of sugar, it didn't seem to slow its consumption.

CHAPTER 3

From the Raj to Uncle Sam

Sugar Daddies

A *New* New World

S UGAR-INDUCED UPHEAVAL continued to affect whole populations of people — some by deception, some at gunpoint.

European-owned sugarcane plantations in Africa began to take root along the southeastern shore of the continent and the islands just outside. Madagascar, Mauritius and Réunion had all been colonized by Dutch, French, or British forces as early as the 1600s — or sometimes all three in succession. But with slavery made illegal, plantation owners needed to find a new source of (preferably cheap) labor.

India, though it stood as the birthplace of refined sugar more than 2,000 years earlier, received little attention for sugar production during the high years of colonialism in the Americas. But as cane cultivation developed in Africa, India was becoming increasingly colonized under the British Raj. In the years following the abolishment of slavery in the British colonies in 1834, Indian sugar exports increased significantly — up to 66,000 tons per year.[17] But otherwise, the country was in rough shape. Crop failure, famine, poverty, and unemployment grew rampant. People became desperate for work of any kind.

And colonists abroad were desperate for *workers* of any kind. British business and tradesmen between India, Africa, England, and the Americas soon developed a system that worked to their advantage: large supplies of laborers from India could be contracted to work on sugarcane plantations across the ocean for a prolonged, but defined, period of time — anywhere from three to ten years. In exchange, employers promised room, board, and transportation to and from the work site. Because workers were guaranteed a return voyage home and usually allotted a small stipend, it couldn't be considered slavery — on paper, anyway. In practice, it became hard to tell the difference.

Between 1835 and 1917, more than one million Indian people set sail for work on the sugar and crop plantations in the Caribbean and Africa; more than three-quarters of them would never return home.[18] Upon arrival at their work stations, the laborers were informed that they were indebted to the company for the costs of their meals, lodging, transportation, and work equipment. They could not leave the plantation until their debts were paid in full. In this sense, they were more like slaves than contracted workers, forced under penalty of law and punishment to toil under harsh conditions for little monetary reward.

Gandhi in Natal

More than 150,000 indentured laborers from India wound up in Natal, on the eastern coast of modern-day South Africa. As in the Caribbean and American plantations, the amount of sugarcane field and mill workers greatly outnumbered the amount of owners, yet all social and political power remained in the hands of the European colonialists.

Indians in Africa were treated in much the same way Africans had been in the New World; ironically, Europeans were wary of enslaving "wild" Africans in their own land. Still, both were subjugated to severe racial oppression, forced to ride in separate car trains from whites or required to carry a note from their employers to walk the streets at night. Even then, they were forbidden from using the sidewalks.

Such was the climate in Natal in 1893 when Mohandas Gandhi, then a 24-year-old London-educated barrister-at-law, arrived to work as a legal liaison for a local trading company. Despite his education, position, and smart style of English dress, Gandhi endured the same kind of humiliating and degrading discrimination as any indentured servant or slave.

After a year of working for the trading company, Gandhi elected to remain in Africa to work as an advocate for social justice on the behalf of sugar plantation workers throughout southern Africa. He organized mass demonstrations and political protests in Natal and Johannesburg, gradually developing the philosophy of nonviolent resistance that would characterize his work for the rest of his life.

Gandhi remained in Africa for twenty more years before returning to India to become a leading national figure in the movement for independence from Great Britain. His work has inspired civil rights causes around the world, and just like the revolutions in the U.S., Haiti, and France, it all started with a little sugar.

U.S. Sugar After Slavery

While many indentured servants from India also worked in the Caribbean and Central and South America, their numbers alone could not supply the tremendous amount of labor required for global sugar production. They were joined by workers in similar situations from impoverished countries such as China, Japan, and the Philippines.

In the United States, beet farming had taken off in the Pacific Northwest to supply more domestic sugar. The fields there were mainly staffed by low-paid Japanese workers, a practice that continued all the way through World War II with the use of forced labor in the internment camps that kept Japanese-Americans socially and racially segregated from the rest of the country.

The labor shortage was particularly severe in the American South with the emancipation of slaves after the Civil War. As in the Caribbean and Africa, plantation owners developed a system that limited workers' rights, freedoms, liberties, and ability to make a living wage while not technically "slavery" in the eyes of the law. Well through the 1940s, the Black Codes in the South kept African-Americans in a perpetual debt peonage system without the right to own property or land. Freedpeople on the streets were assumed to be vagrants or deserters and could be fined and jailed — or sent to involuntary labor camps to keep sugar production running.

As the United States continued to expand, trade over the Pacific Ocean became increasingly important to the U.S. economy. Chief among the list of goods coming in from the Pacific was, of course, sugar.

An American Coup

The archipelago of Hawaii is where the two stories of sugar converge. The first is of the natural expansion of sugarcane as a domesticated crop, which had spread from its original birthplace in New Guinea and was cultivated in the Hawaiian Islands since at least the 7th century CE. As in other Asian and Pacific islands, the sugarcane in Hawaii was valued by the indigenous people as a calorie- and nutrient-dense food. Refining technologies would not make it to the islands for another thousand years or more; cane was always chewed whole, so its many nutrients and fiber were consumed.

The second story is that of sugar colonization. When Christian missionaries from the U.S. first arrived in Hawaii in the 1820s and saw fields of sugarcane, they no doubt recognized the potential for establishing a refined sugar industry on the islands. Many stayed on beyond their Christian duties to construct large-scale mills and plantations that could refine sugar for direct trade with the United States. By the 1860s, the fertile land of Hawaii was so overrun with sugarcane that author Mark Twain dubbed the nation "the king of the sugar world, as far as astonishing productiveness is concerned."[19]

Businesses took notice. Five companies emerged as the dominant players in sugar production and trade, all founded by American expats: Alexander & Baldwin, C. Brewer & Co., Theo H. Davies & Co., American Factors, and Castle & Cooke — the last of which went on to merge with the Hawaiian

Pineapple Company, founded by fellow American James Dole. Together, the two formed the world's largest fruit and vegetable company to this day, Dole Foods.

Instead of fighting each other as competitors, the "Big Five" sugar companies cooperated and bonded in an effort to strengthen Hawaii's ties with the American economy and enact considerable influence over the local Hawaiian government and policymaking. In 1876, the U.S. and the Kingdom of Hawaii managed a reciprocity treaty that granted Hawaiian sugar duty-free importation into the U.S. and gave America rights to establish a military naval base on Oahu in Pu'u Loa, also known as Pearl Harbor.

The more wealth the Hawaiian-American sugar business amassed for the islands, the more the kingdom grew dependent on cane for its economy. Sugar barons gained an increasing influence over local politics, and the native monarchy struggled to maintain authority over the islands.

In 1887, a group of businessmen, most of them American sugar plantation owners, held Hawaiian King Kalākaua at gunpoint until he signed and accepted the terms of a new constitution (which came to be called the Bayonet Constitution, for obvious reasons) that effectively reduced the power of the throne, increased the political rights of American citizens residing in Hawaii, and minimized the power of the native people. Hawaii became a corporatocracy, a nation governed by corporate sugar interests, with the king as a mere figurehead.

When the crown passed from Kalākaua to his sister Lili'uokalani after his death in 1891, the new Queen attempted to re-strengthen the power of the monarchy and the native Hawaiian people. But on January 17, 1893, seven men — five Americans and two Europeans — staged a *coup d'etat* forcing Lili'uokalani to abdicate the throne under threat of violence and war. Following the Queen's arrest and confinement, the wealthy landowners of the islands established a provisional government with Sanford Dole, cousin of pineapple king James Dole, as acting president.

The new rulers of Hawaii immediately petitioned for annexation of the islands by the American government.

President Grover Cleveland, however, saw things differently. He condemned the Hawaiian coup as "an act of war" that was "wholly without justification" and called for the immediate reinstatement of Queen Lili'uokalani. Cleveland testified to Congress that "a substantial wrong has thus been done which... we should endeavor to repair,"[20] and he refused to acknowledge the legitimacy of the new government.

Nonetheless, the provisional Republic of Hawaii remained firmly in place for another four years — just long enough for Cleveland's term as President to draw to a close. Under William McKinley's presidency, Hawaii became an official territory of the United States, in July 1898.

Meanwhile, in Cuba...

Cuba was enjoying a golden age of sugar production while still under Spanish colonial rule. The Haitian Rebellion in the eastern part of Hispaniola had quickly spread west, and many colonists fled the island and took their sugar business elsewhere. By the mid-19th century, Cuba and its sister Spanish colony Puerto Rico were the only islands in the Caribbean that still allowed the use of slave labor, so costs of production on those islands remained much cheaper than in other colonies. By the 1870s, Cuba produced 41% of the world's sugar supply — more than 700,000 tons a year.[21]

By the time slavery was abolished in Cuba in 1886, cane dominated the landscape — so much so that food crops and livestock were all displaced by sugarcane plantations; the island had to import practically everything for survival — especially, and ironically, food. The entire economy of Cuba balanced precipitously on the success of a single commodity: sugar.

As in Hawaii, the Cuban sugar industry was aided by American businessmen. The United States imported as much as 82% of Cuba's sugar product every year and provided many basic goods in return. But Cuba remained a colony of the Spanish, hampered by tariffs and trade restrictions. Multiple attempts at revolution in Cuba were quashed by Spanish forces. But with the help of their powerful U.S. neighbor, Cubans thought independence could be in reach. The United States, however, refused to intervene — until something unexpected forced its hand.

"Remember the Maine, to Hell with Spain!"

On February 15, 1898, the USS *Maine*, an American ship docked in the harbor of Havana, suddenly exploded. To this day, it's unclear who or what caused the combustion, but popular opinion swayed by sensationalist journalism in the United States roundly blamed Spain, and President McKinley was pressed to declare war over the incident.

The ensuing Spanish-American War officially lasted all of ten weeks. Theodore Roosevelt famously proclaimed it a "splendid little war," and its effects on the western hemisphere were great. With its defeat, Spain relinquished control over its last vestiges from the colonial era. Cuba was granted its independence, while Puerto Rico, Guam, and the Philippines were handed over to the United States and became official territories.

American economic and political influence escalated greatly in the years following Cuba's independence. The 1901 Platt Amendment allowed for almost unlimited U.S. intervention in Cuban affairs, barring official annexation. By 1905, 10% of all land in Cuba — more than 4,000 square miles — belonged to American citizens, much of it devoted to growing or refining sugarcane. By the 1950s, Americans owned more than 10,000 square miles of Cuba. And the world market for sugar had continued to expand in the first half of the 20th century, as consumer markets expanded and opened in new and developing countries all over the globe.

Cuba's economy remained at the mercy of the international sugar trade. Global competition, inclement weather, two World Wars, devastating hurricanes, and the unpredictable flux of the price of sugar flung Cuba through vacillating periods of tremendous wealth and prosperity offset by episodes of scarcity and hardship.

Ripe for Revolution

The government of Cuba often acted blindly in the interests of sugar at the expense of the real needs of its people. Corrupt officials conspired heavily with U.S. investors, and a string of dictatorial leaders in Cuba restricted the rights and freedoms of the common people.

Fidel Castro was born on his family's sugar plantation in 1926. By 1959, he had led the overthrow of the government in the Cuban Revolution and assumed power. His nationalization of the sugar industry, his overt contempt of American influence over Cuban affairs, and his growing alliances with the communist Soviet Union put a heavy strain on Cuban-American relations. In July of 1960, President Eisenhower signed into law a bill forbidding the purchase of Cuban-made sugar — the first act in a long line of economic sanctions and embargoes against Cuba that remained largely in effect for over half a century; only in 2015 have diplomatic relations between the two countries begun to shift.

In defiance, Cuba turned instead to a prosperous trade relationship with the USSR. The Soviets, instead of the Americans, now imported roughly 80% of Cuba's sugar crop and provided food and materials in return.

When the USSR collapsed in 1991, most of its trade with Cuba fell with it. Cuba's economy took a hard nosedive. Since then, half of the country's sugar mills have closed, and poverty plagues the Cuban people still.[22]

Modern Big Sugar

Alfonso Fanjul, Jr., was only 21 when the communist revolutionaries of Fidel Castro's new Cuba confiscated all of his family's sugar plantations and mills. The Fanjuls, descended from Spanish colonists, were well established in the Cuban sugar business, with more than 150,000 acres of cane and ten refining mills. But their home, a palatial European-style estate, and all of its possessions were confiscated, nationalized, and later converted into the Museo Nacional de Bellas Artes de Cuba. In the early 1960s, the Fanjul family, along with thousands of other Cubans, fled to the United States.

At the time, Florida had only minimal sugar agriculture. But the Fanjul family was eager to start back up in the trade. Patriarch Alfonso, Sr., bought 4,000 acres of land near Lake Okeechobee in southern Florida and with sons Alfy Jr., Pepe, Alexander, and Andres, founded an entirely new American sugar empire.

Today, the Fanjul Corporation owns such brand names as Domino Sugar, Florida Crystals, C&H Sugar, Redpath Sugar, and Tate & Lyle European Sugar. It operates ten refineries and four mills between six different countries — including the world's largest sugar mill in the Dominican Republic — producing a combined six million tons of sugar a year.[23]

Sugarcane is still the most-planted crop in the world. There's more sugarcane in the world than the next two leading crops — corn and wheat — combined.[24] And every ounce of sugar produced is sold. Almost 63 million tons of sugar circulated the globe in 2014, much of it embedded in the foods we buy off the shelves.[25]

Modern in Some Ways

Despite improvements in farming, it is estimated that half of the world's sugarcane is still harvested by hand, and it is still some of the most difficult manual labor there is.

Harvesting cane manually tends to produce more efficient cuts with less waste than using mechanical means, but the price of human costs is grave. In 2013, the U.S. Department of Labor cited human rights violations in Belize, Bolivia, Brazil, Burma, Colombia, the Dominican Republic, El Salvador, Guatemala, Kenya, Mexico, Pakistan, Panama, Paraguay, the Philippines, Thailand, and Uganda for the use of either child labor or forced labor in sugarcane production.[26]

In Brazil, where more than 1.1 million people are employed in the sugar industry, government raids of plantations in rural areas near the Amazon rainforest in just one year freed more than 4,500 people from "modern-day slavery," though estimates suggest tens if not hundreds of thousands more remain.[27]

"Run from cutting cane any way you can," a former Brazilian worker told a journalist for the *New York Times*; "it is the surest way of being a slave without even knowing it."[28]

Documentary films including *Big Sugar* and *The Price of Sugar* depict harrowing scenes of the modern cane laborer's life: overcrowded and dilapidated shacks, minimal food and water supplies, lack of access to medical attention, and the constant threat of deportation for migrant workers — Jamaicans in the United States, Haitians in the Dominican Republic. A 2011 independent third-party report commissioned by the Coca-Cola Company found that in the Dominican Republic, "regular access to potable water is still a challenge in *bateys*," the camps where workers live. It also found that "families of 5-10 still crowd into small 1-2 room houses," and that proper sanitation systems, electricity, and education for children of workers is severely limited.[29] The United States, however, remains the biggest buyer of Dominican sugar.

The Same Old Problem

In other words, over the five centuries since Christopher Columbus first brought sugarcane to the New World, not much has changed in the quest for sugar. The coupling of sugar and slavery has merely bounced from island to island and continent to continent. The master-slave dynamic that shaped the cane fields of the western hemisphere still persists today.

The global food system actually depends on sugar as a source of calories to feed the world population. Without sugar, we likely wouldn't have enough calories to sustain all human life on earth. Sugar packs a lot of edible calories into every small bite, making it a seemingly efficient way to provide food for many.

But as history has shown, it has come at a terrible price. It's remarkable to realize how political relations and whole cultures have been shaped and shrouded by a food as seemingly innocuous as sugar. No less than five revolutionary wars in the modern world have sprung from the injustices of sugar production. Cuba, as we saw, is a poignant example of how the power and influence of sugar can make or break an entire nation.

The next example, the United States, shows how sugar can infiltrate an entire nation's diet. It's proof that, while people used to control sugar production, now the sugar controls us.

PART II:

The American Diet Revolution

How Sugar Invaded Our Country

CHAPTER 4

Cocaine & Corn Flakes

Diseases of War

JOHN STITH PEMBERTON WAS a licensed pharmacist, a veteran of the Confederate Army, a morphine addict, and the inventor of Coca-Cola.

After he was slashed across the chest during the last battle of the Civil War in his native Georgia, Pemberton was, like many of his generation, prescribed morphine for the pain — which, of course, turned out to be highly addictive. Yet by the 1890s, the opium-derived drug was a popular American cure-all for everything from infants' teething pain to morning sickness. It was also used to treat adult-onset diabetes, which had become catastrophically more prevalent after the Civil War.

Dr. Richard Thomas Williamson, a British field doctor who wrote an 1898 book on the subject, claimed to have "clearly shown the value of morphine in reducing the amount of sugar in the urine in cases of diabetes" and recommended patients take one grain, or about 60mg, three times a day — "or even larger doses, without any bad effects."[30] (Today, the highest doctor-prescribed morphine dosages are 100mg, but only for patients who have developed a previous tolerance to the substance and are in severe, chronic, or terminal pain.)

Once a rare disease, diabetes was killing Americans at a rate that increased 1500% between 1865 and 1920, even as medical understanding and technology was improving.[31] Around the turn of the 20th century, diabetes had become especially prevalent among upper-class white males and veterans of the Civil War. The ration foods of soldiers on both the Union and Confederate sides typically subsisted of hardtack (a plain, dry cracker), salt beef or pork, and, most importantly, coffee and sugar.

"It was coffee *at* meals and *between* meals," Massachusetts veteran John D. Billings wrote in his popular 1887 memoirs; "men going on guard or coming off guard drank it at all hours of the night, and to-day the old soldiers who can stand it are the hardest coffee-drinkers in the community, through the schooling which they received in the service."[32] Sugar was rationed accordingly with coffee, since "coffee to drink *without* sweetening... was not to [a soldier's] taste."[33]

Coffee in America at the time was almost always served with plenty of milk, too, but since fresh milk would spoil, most soldiers took it in condensed form. Canned condensed milk, invented in the 1850s in upstate New York, was seen as a good, portable food for soldiers on the go. At more than 1,000 calories per seventy-five cent can during the Civil War (including a whopping 200 grams of sugar), sweetened condensed milk was not exactly cheap for the everyday soldier, but it was worth it. To put that into perspective, using conversion rates from the 1860s, that can would cost between $16 and $22 in 2015.

After the Civil War, veterans brought home with them a penchant for sweetened condensed milk, even preferring it over regular fresh milk. Markets continued to expand for the new product, and the price of one of its principal ingredients — sugar — was falling dramatically. Between the 1870s and 1890s, the real cost of sugar fell by 114%.[34] By 1915, per capita consumption of refined white sugar doubled in the United States.[35] In the same time period, rates of diabetes surged.

Snake Oil Cocktails

It wasn't just diabetes that afflicted American eaters; there was a sudden scourge of digestive and intestinal issues that pharmaceutical companies tried to fix with new-fangled medicines, tonics, and drugs. The underlying cause of many stomach problems was probably a poor diet and too much sugar, but no businessman could make a profit selling such common sense.

Instead, the United States saw the rise of the snake oil salesman in the latter part of the 19th century. More often than not, these cure-alls were no more than a concoction of morphine, alcohol, and sugar. The narcotic effects of the drugs provided temporary relief from virtually any ailment, leading consumers to believe that they might actually work.

New drugs appeared on the market all the time: the Bayer Aspirin Company, for example, developed an opium-derived cough suppressant under the brand name Heroin, which was simultaneously marketed as a non-habit-forming morphine alternative. The product was pulled in 1910 when the company recognized that heroin was actually a more potent strain of morphine itself.

French Coca Wine

In the 1860s, scientists in Europe successfully isolated the cocaine alkaloid, the psychoactive part of the coca leaf native to South America. Without much study of its effects, physicians began using it to treat everything from toothaches and anxiety to syphilis and respiratory illness. Esteemed doctors praised cocaine for "its marked tonic effect upon the heart, nervous system and capillaries, and its power to invigorate the system, to improve nutrition, and to sustain life."[36]

In 1863, a French chemist named Angelo Mariani began bottling cocaine mixed with Bordeaux wine. Mariani pushed his Vin Mariani drink as a health tonic and intellectual stimulant, augmenting the drink's reputation by sending complimentary samples to celebrities and public figures of the day; Thomas Edison, Sir Arthur Conan Doyle, President William McKinley, Queen

Victoria, and Pope Leo XIII were all said to be great imbibers of the drink, a bottle of which contained up to 140mg of cocaine.[37]

Vin Mariani was less widely available in the States than it was in Europe, but its brand and reputation became well known among the intellectual upper classes. John Stith Pemberton, the wounded veteran pharmacist, believed that coca might be the cure to his crippling morphine addiction. In 1884, he set out to brand a drink of his own.

"Pemberton's French Wine Coca" stood apart from the competition with its additional trendy medicinal ingredients: kola nuts, an African fruit with high concentrations of natural caffeine, and damiana, a leaf from the Americas with supposed aphrodisiacal properties. Pemberton's French Wine Coca was, according to local advertisements, "infallible in curing all who are afflicted with any nerve trouble, dyspepsia, mental and physical exhaustion, all chronic and wasting diseases, gastric irritability, constipation, sick headache, neuralgia... seminal weakness, impotency, etc., when all other remedies fail."[38]

Pemberton was met early on with legal challenges to his product. In 1886, several counties in Georgia, including Pemberton's home and the city of Atlanta, went dry. So he set about creating an alcohol-free version of his tonic. Instead of wine, Pemberton used a plain sugar syrup to mask the bitter taste of the medicinal plants and named it after its two remaining principal ingredients, cocaine and kola: Coca-Cola.

Both the alcoholic and Prohibition-friendly versions of the cocaine-infused drink sold well throughout Georgia and other nearby parts of the American south, but Pemberton's health was failing. Still nursing a morphine addiction, he fell ill to stomach cancer and died in 1888, not long after selling the drinks' patent rights to fellow druggist Asa Candler.

The Battle Creek Sanitarium

Not everyone condoned the fad miracle drugs sweeping the nation. In Michigan, a diet and wellness movement based in asceticism and simplicity was founded in direct opposition to the day's deceptive snake-oil tonics. Its leader was Dr. John Harvey Kellogg, chief medical officer and superintendent of the Battle Creek Sanitarium, a sort of precursor to today's luxury health spa resorts. The Sanitarium became a haven for the well-to-do to seek cures for their minor illnesses such as indigestion or stress, and its reputation as an expensive retreat helped foster the popularity of Kellogg's dietary movement.

Kellogg, a devout Seventh-day Adventist, promoted an exiguous vegetarian diet, daily exercise, daily enemas, and plenty of fresh air. Alcohol, meat, eggs, tobacco, salt, and sugar were verboten at the Sanitarium — Dr. Kellogg viewed them as unnecessary additions to an otherwise complete diet of natural grains, fruits, and vegetables.

After their stays at the Sanitarium, many people returning home reported a new sense of health and energy. Many patients returned every few years for a "detox." At its peak, the Sanitarium hosted more than three thousand patients a year, among them Mary Todd Lincoln, Henry Ford, Amelia Earhart, and President William Howard Taft.

If Coca-Cola, French wine coca, and the other drugged-up snake oil tonics were about achieving health and productivity through the stimulation of the senses, the Battle Creek Sanitarium diet was all about minimalism and suppression. The food served was purposely bland and tasteless; common dinner menus included items such as graham grits, gluten gruel, dyspeptic wafers — and for dessert, stewed prunes.

Eating, according to Kellogg, was meant to be functional, not enjoyable. "Exciting stimulants and condiments weaken and irritate [the] nerves and derange the circulation," he wrote in his first book, *Plain Facts for Old and Young.*[39]

The Ready-to-Eat Breakfast Cereal

Despite, or perhaps because of, Kellogg's dreary dietary prescriptions, the meals of Battle Creek Sanitarium began to amass a cult following. All foods were prepared on-site, but converted patrons wanted a way to easily continue their diets at home.

While Dr. John Kellogg preferred keeping his practice within the Sanitarium walls, his younger brother and bookkeeper, William Keith Kellogg, saw an opportunity. The most popular of the Sanitarium's foods were the cereal grains that had been dried and either cut, shredded, or flaked for eating. They were meant to be served plain and uncooked, unlike other commercial cereals. William worked with packaging and distribution companies to bring Toasted Corn Flakes to market in 1897. The association between the Kellogg name and the Battle Creek Sanitarium immediately branded the food as a health-conscious product and bolstered sales among concerned housewives and mothers leery of the typical American breakfast of sausage and eggs.

Fad vs. Fad

The grain and cereal fad served as a direct counter to the health tonic craze sweeping the country. John Kellogg made a point to use his authority to augment his own business while disparaging others. Coca-Cola and other drinks, he claimed, were "an evil... to be suppressed."[40]

"Every scientific physician knows that almost every one of the claims that have been made respecting the virtues of coca wine, no matter of whose make, are stupendously false," the Battle Creek Sanitarium's journal/newsletter, *Modern Medicine and Bacteriological Review*, states. "Whatever other virtues these drugs possess, they certainly do not possess the power to give either health or strength."[41]

The general American pubic soon came to agree with him — at least on the subject of cocaine, which was gradually outlawed throughout the country, beginning with Coca-Cola's home state of Georgia in 1902. Like Pemberton before him, Coca-Cola's new proprietor Asa Candler met legal restrictions by altering the drink's recipe to remove the offending drug while upping the levels of sugar and caffeine in its place to keep customers interested, satisfied, and coming back for more.

The Industrial Food Revolution

Leaps in industrial technology enabled companies like Coca-Cola and Kellogg's to distribute their goods across the country, allowing specific brands of food to become recognized at a national level. The turn of the 20th century was a pivotal period in the rise of giant food processors. Milton Hershey founded his namesake chocolate company in Pennsylvania in 1894; the H.J. Heinz Company already had "57 varieties" to its name by that time. A conglomerate of 114 American bakeries consolidated to form the National Biscuit Company, or Nabisco, in 1898. And the success of Coca-Cola and Kellogg's inspired a legion of imitators, from Pepsi-Cola and RC Cola to Post Cereals and General Mills.

It amounted to a revolution in eating: the industrialization of tasks like baking and canning saved middle-class Americans time and the upper classes the need for servants and cooks. But the manufacturing of ready-made food, while explosively popular, was highly unregulated. As with health tonic drinks, food makers could make any sort of unverified claims on their products; Post's flagship cereal, Grape-Nuts, was sold as a "brain food" purportedly capable of curing malaria, consumption, and loose teeth.[42] Coca-Cola, though its principal ingredients were now only caffeine and sugar, continued to market itself as a health tonic and cure-all.

Food and Fraud

In his 1905 book *The Great American Fraud*, journalist Samuel Hopkins Adams roundly exposed the tonic and patent medicine industry for what it was. The book revealed many popular drugs as mere cocktails of sugar, opiates, caffeine, and cocaine cleverly packaged to persuade consumers that the narcotic effects of the drugs were providing real healing instead of a temporary, drug-induced relief. Coca-Cola was, then and now, the most popular drink in America. Though cocaine had been removed from the formula, Adams still condemned the drink as addictive.

"I do most emphatically believe that [Coca-Cola] produces a habit, not so pronounced, indeed, as alcohol or morphine addiction, but nevertheless, baneful and difficult to break," Adams wrote in a 1907 letter printed in *The Druggists Circular*. "…I hear from all parts of the South, both by letter and personal interview, of cases where the addict must have his fifteen or twenty glasses of 'dope' (the Southern term for coca cola) per day."[43]

The Great American Fraud did to the medicine and beverage industry what Upton Sinclair's *The Jungle*, printed the following year, did to the meat industry. Once consumers knew the truth, they felt betrayed and outraged. With the help of Adams, Sinclair, and support from President Theodore Roosevelt, the 1906 Pure Food and Drug Act passed through Congress, establishing the Bureau of Chemistry (later the Food and Drug Administration) as a government-sanctioned authority to crack down on mislabeled or adulterated foods.

Forty Barrels and Twenty Kegs

The Chief of Staff of the Bureau of Chemistry, Dr. Harvey Wiley, had already proved an immensely influential proponent of consumer rights and advocacy in the burgeoning age of industrialized food. His "Poison Squad" studies in 1902, wherein a group of healthy young men would consume common (and sometimes hazardous) food additives to test their bodily effects, not only popularized the need for food safety and testing but managed to eliminate harmful chemicals such as Borax, sulfuric acid, saltpeter, copper sulfate, and formaldehyde from processed and canned foods.

Wiley was dogmatic in his approach to enforcing "pure" foods. High on his list of potentially suspect additives was caffeine, which was being synthesized and manufactured by chemical companies such as Monsanto and widely used in many beverages. Wiley feared it would "not be long before a milk dealer will discover that by adding a grain or two of caffeine to his milk it will become more popular... and soon we will have our bread and meat treated in the same way."[44]

Coca-Cola used artificial caffeine as a cheaper alternative to kola nuts for the mass production of its fountain syrup, which was selling five million gallons every year. The company roused Wiley's suspicion with its scores of reported Coca-Cola addicts, particularly in its native south. On October 20, 1909, federal government officials seized a shipment of Coca-Cola at the Georgia-Tennessee border. The company was charged with the transportation of misbranded and adulterated goods over state lines — misbranded because the product contained only scant amounts of either coca or kola, adulterated because of the addition of synthesized caffeine.

After a trial and a string of appeals, the case eventually went before the Supreme Court in *United States v. Forty Barrels and Twenty Kegs of Coca-Cola.*

Weeks before the hearings, Coca-Cola hired a psychology instructor, Harry Hollingworth, to conduct human trials on the effects of caffeine. Within forty days, Hollingworth produced three complete studies arguing that caffeine did not affect any motor or cognitive abilities.[45] Hollingworth's testimony was instrumental in winning the case for Coca-Cola and keeping the company alive after seven years of court proceedings.

The *US v. Coca-Cola* case is both pivotal and ironic. Suddenly, science itself could have opinions, depending on what questions were being asked — or, more likely, who was paying the bills. And it's ironic that Dr. Harvey Wiley's prejudices against caffeine and the Coca-Cola Company itself likely sent him chasing down the wrong ingredient. Today, it's not caffeine that's added to our milks, breads, and meats to hook consumers: it's sugar.

Today, seventy percent of all milk sold in school cafeterias is chocolate-flavored and sweetened. Most slices of supermarket white bread contain multiple grams of added sugars. Deli meats are routinely preserved and enhanced with sugar. Sugar (as we'll discuss more in coming chapters) is the highly addictive factor in foods and soft drinks.

The seven-year-long Coke case was exhausting. Wiley resigned from his post in the Bureau of Chemistry before the trial was even over. He actually spent his final years studying sugar chemistry and sorghum, hoping to foster a strong domestic sugar industry in the United States.

According to the *Pennsylvania Medical Journal*, "Dr. Wiley declared he had resigned because almost from the beginning of his service he had been antagonized in the enforcement of the pure food and drug law."[46] Wiley was clearly frustrated by how quickly and easily food companies managed to circumvent governmental regulation, and how willing, in turn, the government was to overlook such tactics. Apart from banning a few poisons and passing a few laws to appease the public, Wiley was unable to enact very much change during his government tenure.

Kellogg v. Kellogg

Back in Michigan, another lengthy series of trials was also shaping the future of food in the United States. In *Kellogg v. Kellogg*, Dr. John Harvey sued his brother William Keith over the use of the Kellogg name on mass-produced cereals such as Toasted Corn Flakes.

Going against his brother's wishes, William, who owned the rights over cereal production, had begun adding sugar to the recipes for Corn Flakes, Wheat Flakes, Rice Flakes, Bran Flakes, and other products of the Kellogg's Company in 1905. The sweeter-tasting cereals had surged in popularity.

Either because he didn't want his name associated with a sugar-adulterated product or because he wanted a better cut of the tremendous profits the cereals were earning, Dr. John Harvey sued Will for illegal appropriation of trade secrets and wrongful use of the name "Kellogg." An out-of-court settlement in 1911 allowed Will to continue using the Kellogg name, but more suits followed: a final decision by the Michigan State Supreme Court in 1920 ruled in favor of William Keith, who continued to market his sugar-enhanced cereals under the Kellogg name.

Siding With Sugar

To this day, Kellogg's and Coca-Cola are two of the most prominent sources of sugar in our diets. One in three Americans start their day, every day, with sweetened breakfast cereals that can contain as much sugar as a Coke itself. Fifty percent of Americans drink at least one sugar-sweetened beverage every day. A single cup serving of Kellogg's Honey Smacks cereal contains 10 grams of sugar, and a twelve-ounce serving of Coke contains 39 grams. Just one of these common foods alone eats up most of the recommended limit of 25 grams of added sugars per day; consuming both in a day would put anybody well over what is considered the reasonable sugar threshold.

Both started off as health products to cure ailing Americans, yet both created a host of new problems by pushing sugar to turn profits. Today, their brand images remain linked to ideas of well-being and healthy living. Coke posits itself as essentially a national pastime, a deserved moment of relaxation and pleasure. Kellogg's promotes children's health and growth while simultaneously marketing the most sugary cereals directly at youth during TV cartoons. Are these images any more or less false and misleading than the tonics and cure-alls from the golden age of the snake oil salesman?

Since its early first attempts with the Pure Food and Drug Act, the government has been thwarted by the food companies in trying to control the food market. Since there are policies in place by the government that allow for the putting of addictive and harmful products like sugar in foods — and it's not the fault of the food companies that sugar is addictive — they can't be held directly responsible, even as overconsumption of these "safe" products brings enormous health and economic costs to our society.

CHAPTER 5

A Growing Problem

A PERFECT STORM OF ECONOMIC RECESSION, runaway inflation, crop failures, and an international energy crisis made the 1970s a particularly festering hotbed for American food politics. Prices of basic nutritive staples like grains and beef were in constant flux, sending consumers and food manufacturers into a panic. The price of sugar was especially volatile: in late 1973, a pound on the world market cost ten cents. Just a year later, the price had more than quintupled to 57 cents per pound. The Nixon Administration, and especially Secretary of Agriculture Earl Butz, was under tremendous pressure to calm and stabilize the cost of food and ensure the proper feeding of the nation.

You might say Nixon and Butz solved the food crisis too well. Today, the U.S. food economy produces 500 more calories per person per day than it did in the 1970s, and the average American puts away 200 calories more than they did then.[47] Not that it costs us anything extra: through most of the 1970s, Americans spent nearly 14% of their personal income on food expenditures; today that figure is less than 10%. In fact, Americans spend less of their money on food than any other country in the world.[48] Together, the farm economy and food manufacturers are able to produce a litany of consumable goods from just a few choice ingredients — especially corn.

Secretary Earl Butz's legacy is in completely overturning the forty years of agricultural policy that preceded him. Since the New Deal programs of Franklin Roosevelt, American farmers were prescribed careful production quotas to help keep the price of crops steady and secure. The system worked, but the country wasn't producing enough food to feed itself: part of the reason for the food price frenzy of the 1970s was America's dependence on imported goods. So Butz, himself from a line of Indiana dairy farmers, encouraged American farmers to grow as much as they could — to "get big or get out" — and the farmers listened and started producing.

Corn is one of the most efficient crops to grow on the vast expanse of soil in the American Midwest. Farmers were now given free rein to produce as much as possible. And selective breeding and genetic engineering through the years produced varieties of corn that were able to produce larger ears, with more kernels of corn per ear. Stalks could be grown taller, closer together, and more quickly with the help of chemical fertilizers developed after World War II. Today, one acre of corn yields four times the amount of calories it could only fifty years ago.

However, the vast majority is not the same as the maize that Native Americans ate for millennia, or even what's for sale at markets all summer long. Less than one percent of all corn grown in the United States is even edible straight from the stalk. The rest — over 95 million acres' worth — is a special variety called dent corn, which has been engineered to contain much higher amounts of starch. Dent corn can be harvested and processed into myriad types of food and fuel. Forty percent is converted into ethanol for fuel; another 36% goes toward animal feed, which in turn helps minimize the production costs of meat, poultry, dairy, and even fish that are quickly fattened on a corn-heavy diet. The rest is processed into corn-based foods, ingredients, and preservatives that sweeten, enhance, and bulk up the food products in every grocery store in America. Today, it's estimated that one out of every four items in the typical supermarket contains corn of some kind.[49]

Secretary Butz's push for more large-scale production worked so well that manufacturers and policy-makers were soon looking for more ways to use the surplus. Butz personally flew to Japan to look into a new technology to convert glucose — the building block of starches so abundant in dent corn — into fructose, a sweet simple sugar. Together, glucose and fructose bind in nature to form sucrose, what we know as common table sugar. Japanese scientists had been working for more than a dozen years to alter the chemical structure of glucose to convert it into fructose, its sweeter and more delicious counterpart. Finally, in 1970, they were able to produce a dissolvable liquid whose sweetness could be controlled. They set the balance at roughly 55% fructose to 45% glucose to mimic the sweetness of cane or beet sugar, and high-fructose corn syrup was born.

The United States quickly adopted the technology, using corn as the starchy base, and soon high-fructose corn syrup (HFCS) flooded the American food market. Its advantages were many: high-fructose corn syrup is significantly cheaper to produce than traditional sugar, and while cane and beet sugar farms are well represented on American soil, they could never satisfy the needs of the entire nation. Supplementing the sweets market with corn-derived syrup also allowed the U.S. to decrease its foreign sugar imports and become increasingly self-reliant.

Corn production is much less labor-intensive than cane or beets, lessening the dependency on low-paid and migrant workers. As a liquid, high-fructose corn syrup does not need to be first dissolved, like sugar, to use in food and beverage products. It significantly increases the shelf life of baked goods as compared with sugar, which attracts moisture. HFCS also has a lower freezing point than liquid sugar, making it ideal for certain drinks or fruit juice concentrates. It also produces a more instantaneous sensation of sweet perception on the tongue, which, while still distinctive from the taste of sugar, allows the true flavors of other ingredients to shine through.

Gradually, many food manufacturing companies made the nearly imperceptible switch from sugar to HFCS. Soft drink companies such as Coca-Cola and Pepsi were more resistant; as the principal ingredient in most of their products, sugar was perceived as integral to their recipes. But a string of hurricanes in the early 1980s knocked Caribbean sugar production to disastrous lows, and world sugar prices skyrocketed. In 1984, Coca-Cola was the first major beverage company to formally switch U.S. domestic soda production from sugar to HFCS; most others quickly followed suit. Today, about 6% of the 95 million acres of dent corn are specifically for the production of high-fructose corn syrup, of which 70% winds up in some kind of drink.

Fructose by Any Other Name

When researchers try to pinpoint the beginnings of the modern obesity epidemic — over 33% of Americans are currently obese, and another 33% are overweight — they inevitably point to the 1970s. Still, so many rapid changes were taking place in the ways we grow, produce, manufacture, and eat food that a particular cause is difficult to isolate. Yet high-fructose corn syrup, which was never used before the 1970s and has been used in vast quantities ever since, has emerged as public enemy number one in the current battle against obesity. After several medical journal articles probed the potential link between high-fructose corn syrup and obesity in the early 2000s, popular media promptly latched on to the correlation, vilifying HFCS as the principal — and only — cause of obesity. Unfortunately, it's not that simple.

While there are minute chemical and structural differences between high-fructose corn syrup and its inspirational model, sucrose, the way the body metabolizes them is essentially identical. The "high" of high-fructose corn syrup is merely a relative term: most HFCS is 55% fructose to 45% glucose, whereas sucrose is an evenly split 50-50. In chemical composition, HFCS possibly bears more resemblance to nature's only true sweetener, honey, than it does to refined sugar. It's true that over time (and at our mass rates of consumption) biological differences may occur: in just one year, a daily habit of a twenty-ounce soft drink sweetened with HFCS instead of sucrose delivers 730 extra grams of fructose, which is considered to be worse for our health than glucose (more on this in Part III). However, we don't eat HFCS in isolation, and even though rates of its consumption have been declining for a dozen years, our rates of obesity show no signs of slowing.

Packaging labels that boast "Made with Real Sugar" or "No High-Fructose Corn Syrup" are presented as health claims, and consumers are eating it up. Sales of products labeled "No HFCS" had surpassed $1 billion by 2005.[50] But HFCS did not simply replace all sugar, thereby causing obesity — far from it. The consumption of high-fructose corn syrup has never surpassed that of refined sugar in the United States (though in one year, 2003, the amounts were equal). In fact, high-fructose corn syrup barely curtailed our sugar consumption at all: per capita sugar use fell after the initial introduction of HFCS, from 1973 through 1986, but then began to rise again alongside the use of it. High-fructose corn syrup simply made sweets cheaper and much more prevalent in our food system. Consequently, we eat more of both sweeteners than we ever would have when we had only sugar.

The obesity epidemic, of course, is not confined to the United States alone. Worldwide rates of obesity have doubled since 1980, and there are now more overweight than underweight people living around the globe. Yet the United States remains the only country where high-fructose corn syrup makes up a significant portion of the sweetener market; its use around the world is less than 10% of all sugar consumption. The United States remains the most obese country in the world, but the two most populous countries — China and India — have very low rates of high-fructose corn syrup consumption but increasingly higher rates of refined sugar consumption and obesity.[51] Whether it's from cane, beets, or corn, the body doesn't discriminate against sugars of any kind.

Nonetheless, sales and production of high-fructose corn syrup have suffered from years of bad press. Food and drink manufacturers, from Pizza Hut to Snapple Tea, have increasingly switched back to using only refined sugar for the appearance of using "natural" products. But remember: cane and beet sugar must also be extracted, boiled, refined, and processed into pure sucrose; it's not exactly a "natural" process. Except for the harmless enzymatic process that converts glucose molecules into fructose, sweeteners made from corn (or, in other parts of the world, wheat, rice, and cassava) are arguably no more or less naturally occurring than sugars. They all come from plants, but there's a lot of processing and synthesizing involved to get from plant to pure sweetness.

Sweetness on Trial

In 2008, the Corn Refiners Association (CRA) — a conglomerate special interest group representing the nation's largest manufacturers of high-fructose corn syrup, including Archer Daniels Midland, Cargill, and others — launched a $30 million public relations campaign supposedly designed to "provide consumers with credible, science-based information to enable them to make informed decisions about including HFCS in their diet."[52] The aim was to reverse the negative public image of high-fructose corn syrup by touting it as a naturally derived sweetener metabolically and nutritionally equivalent to sugar. The strategy went so far as to petition the FDA to allow the use of the phrase "corn sugar" instead of "high-fructose corn syrup" on ingredient and packaging labels. The petition was denied; however, the FDA stated they "would not object" to the CRA's use of the word "natural" to promote products containing high-fructose corn syrup.[53]

Naturally, sugar producers and manufacturers were not pleased. The vilification of high-fructose corn syrup was good for the sugar business. In April 2011, the Sugar Association (SA) — the sugar industry's equivalent of the CRA — filed a federal lawsuit against the Corn Refiners Association, claiming that the marketing campaign equating HFCS with sugar was false and misleading. The corn companies fired back with a countersuit, accusing the Sugar Association of "deceiving customers into believing that processed sugar is safer and more healthful than high-fructose corn syrup, despite overwhelming scientific evidence that the two forms of sugar are nutritionally equivalent."[54]

The ensuing litigations — still ongoing at the time of this writing as of January 2015 — have revealed eye-opening accounts of what both parties have done to curry and influence public favor. Internal memos from the Sugar

Association in 2004, for example, congratulate itself for feeding "the media with the science to help fuel the public concern and debate on High Fructose Corn Syrup" by funding research that emphasizes the differences between HFCS and sugar and casting HFCS as more insidious. The studies were, even by the group's own standards, flawed — but were published and promoted anyway. [55]

As the Corn Refiners have claimed, other documents from the Sugar Association explicitly state the replacement of HFCS with sugar in the food and beverage sector as one of the organization's top priorities. The CRA, to its credit, acknowledges in its counterclaim that "...vilifying one kind of added sugar will not reduce Americans' waistlines. Reducing all added sugars, and reducing caloric intake in general, will.... The Sugar Association has worked to perpetuate the myth that HFCS uniquely contributes to obesity and other health problems, preying on consumers' fears and diverting attention away from the real issue — that Americans should reduce their consumption of all added sugars and calories in general."[56]

Yet, since 2011, the Corn Refiners Association has spent half a million dollars funding thirty studies from a single research lab in Florida that works to produce scientific evidence of the similarities between HFCS and sugar. Another $3.2 million has gone towards a veiled nonprofit advocacy group, the Center for Consumer Freedom, which lobbies governmental officials and policymakers on behalf of the industry. But these ploys are merely pages taken from the Sugar Association's own book: the group has published and promoted scientific reports that, by the group's own admittance, were flawed and dubious in integrity.[57] The Sugar Association, meanwhile, has donated over half a million dollars over the years to its own Washington consumer advocacy group, Citizens for Health, which in turn has petitioned the FDA for stricter and more transparent labeling practices on items containing high-fructose corn syrup.

Pawns in Their Game

The litigations between the Sugar and Corn Refiners associations speak volumes about the ways consumers are often unwittingly persuaded to like or spurn a given commodity. Of course, all industries, from beef to cigarettes to oil, have their own brand of lobbying tactics. The Sugar Association was originally founded in the late 1940s, just after the end of World War II. During the war, sugar was the first food to be rationed among civilians; each family was allotted two pounds per person per month, about half of the average intake at the time, and restaurant supplies were vastly diminished as well. Government-distributed pamphlets and propaganda encouraged sugar abstinence as a noble cause and patriotic duty.

By the end of the war, sugar consumption was at historic lows and remained that way for a time even after rations were lifted; apparently, Americans had in fact learned to live with less sugar. Quickly, the newly formed Sugar Association set to work, developing marketing and advertising campaigns to bring sugar back to the forefront of the American plate. It even established the Sugar Research Foundation, an industry-funded laboratory that sought to dispel "misconceptions concerning the causes of tooth decay, diabetes, and heart problems."[58]

Through the 1950s and 1960s, the Sugar Association augmented its public relations campaign with advertisements that actually suggested sugar as a diet tool ("Spoil your appetite with sugar, and you could come up with willpower — the willpower you need to eat less, and maybe even weigh less"[59]) and as an important source of energy for children ("Note to Mothers: ...Play safe with your young ones — make sure they get sugar every day"[60]). The Federal Trade Commission ordered the Sugar Association to cease production of these misleading advertisements in 1972, but that hardly put an end to the group's overall efforts; in 1976, they were awarded the highest honor from the Public Relations Society of America, for excellence in "the forging of public opinion."[61]

Sugar lobby interests continue to influence policymaking and governmental regulations today. When the USDA and the Department of Health and

Human Services set out to revise the *Dietary Guidelines for Americans* in 2000, lobbyists rallied thirty senators — half of whom represented cane- or beet-growing states — to prevent the Departments from changing the 1995 guidelines, "Choose a diet moderate in sugars," to the proposed revision advising consumers to "limit sugar intake." The 2000 *Dietary Guidelines* remained unchanged.[62]

Worldwide, the average consumption of added sugars has continued to increase since 1962.[63] Many of those calories come in the form of soft drinks and sweetened beverages. How did that happen? One good example is that the Coca-Cola Company was exempt from WWII sugar rationing in light of its pledge "to see that every man in uniform gets a bottle of Coca-Cola for 5 cents, wherever he is and whatever it costs the Company."[64] With help from the U.S. government, Coke established 64 bottling plants across Europe during wartime. That helped get Coke to American men in uniform, but also allowed the company to introduce its product to entirely new demographics in entirely new countries around the world. Some five billion bottles of Coke were consumed by U.S. troops during the war, and afterwards many returned home with a new penchant for soft drinks: between 1945 and 1975, American consumption of carbonated soft drinks tripled.[65]

And the soft drink market in developing countries continues to soar: both Thailand and Turkey have doubled their consumption rates of Coca-Cola products within the last ten years; Panama has quintupled its intake in the past twenty. Mexico, which now consumes an annual 745 servings of Coke products per person, has become the company's leading customer.[66]

Ironically enough, Mexican Coke has become a coveted commodity in the United States; it's made using refined cane sugar, while the American-made drinks use high-fructose corn syrup. Whatever the taste differences, that Coke is still a Coke and the sugars inside are still sugars. And in recent years, Mexico has given the United States substantial competition for the title of most obese country in the world.

Wrong answers

For most consumers, the battle between sugar and high-fructose corn syrup has gone largely unnoticed — except at the checkout line. The introduction of corn syrup and corn products in the American food market has helped reduce our grocery bills; average food expenses as a percent of income have decreased by 50% since the 1950s, in part because of those corn products.

But they certainly haven't reduced our waistlines — or, for that matter, our health-care spending. In that same timespan, government spending on health-care quadrupled.[67]

Americans, meanwhile, had been concerned about those expanding waistlines for decades.

Once again, the country went searching for answers to its health problems. And once again, we chose the wrong villain — with catastrophic results.

CHAPTER 6

Calories: Sugar vs. Fat

"COUNTING CALORIES NOWADAYS?" A 1950s Domino Sugar magazine advertisement asks. "You should know that generous amounts of Domino Granulated Sugar, used in your favorite foods and beverages, *contain fewer calories* than usual servings of many foods regularly included in reducing diets." Different takes on the ad compare three teaspoons of white sugar to culprits of higher caloric content: a medium-sized apple, half a grapefruit, three tomatoes. "Nutritionists say that *no single* food is fattening unless you take in more calories than your body uses up. Tomatoes, grapefruit, and apples are excellent foods... but sugar, too, is nutritionally important in the well-balanced diet you need for good health."[68]

What the ad says is true: sugar contains about 15 calories per teaspoon, while a tomato has nearly 20, half a grapefruit might have 50, and an apple might have nearly 100. And by oversimplifying the issue to calories, the advertisers were speaking the language of the times.

When chemist Wilbur Olin Atwater (later an agent for the USDA) established the scientific quantification of a calorie as a standard unit of energy in 1894, Americans began to think about food differently.

At first, measuring the calorie contents of foods was a way to help people make cost-effective choices at the grocery store. By comparing the caloric value and cost of foods — pork and chicken, for example — consumers could make more informed decisions. In today's prices, pork chops might cost five or six dollars per pound, which in turn buys 775 calories of pork. Chicken breast, on the other hand, might only cost $3 per pound for 1,000 calories per pound. Thus, every dollar of chicken breast buys more than 300 calories of food, while every dollar of pork buys only about 150 — so chicken offers more food energy for the money. At the dawn of the 20th century, this kind of number-crunching was instrumental in helping low-income families feed their loved ones and also in establishing school lunch programs and balanced nutrition practices.

Within a few short decades, however, the use of calorie-counting had been turned on its head: many Americans, especially women, were using the numbers to forge a mathematic plan for weight loss. By creating a caloric deficit — expending more calories than you consume — one should, by logic, reduce body mass. This straightforward, simple formula has been the basis for thousands of diets and weight-loss programs ever since. It's the standard defense that any food company gives if nutritionists try to pin blame for the obesity epidemic on any singular item, especially sugar. It's what allows companies like Domino Sugar to run ads pitting sugar's calories against those of fruits and vegetables. "We… believe that balance or 'calories in, calories out' must remain the central tenet of achieving weight management and a healthy lifestyle," Kellogg's said in a statement defending the high sugar content of some of their children's cereals.[69]

By this thinking, it doesn't matter where the calories come from, so long as they remain in check. But the "calorie is a calorie" logic leaves out the other vital principal of Wilbur Atwater's analysis: the nutritive value of a food. Clearly, a breakfast that consists of half a grapefruit, a medium apple, and three small tomatoes is going to provide more satiety, more vitamins, fiber, minerals, and physical nourishment than a meal made up solely of nine teaspoons of sugar (which, incidentally, is about the amount of sugar in a Starbucks mocha frappuccino).

So are all calories truly created equal? Each calorie from an apple comes packaged with fiber, B and C vitamins, potassium, calcium, and iron. Calories from refined sugars are just that: calories. They have no nutritive properties, no added value except for their taste appeal. Mankind cannot live off of refined sugar alone, no matter how many calories of it we consume. That's why calories from refined sugar are often called "empty" calories: *there's nothing to them but chemical energy, which is not necessarily the same thing as physical or mental energy.* Without the proper nutrients that come from vitamins, minerals, lipids, and proteins, the body and the mind cannot possibly function.

Refined sugar has no redeeming nutritional qualities. If we eat sugars on top of a fulfilling and balanced diet, we risk consuming excess calories that the body has no use for and stores as fat; if we eat sugars instead of other foods, even when strictly monitoring caloric intake and expenditure, we risk depriving our bodies of the necessary amount of other food qualities it needs. Food cannot be summed up by its calories alone; in effect, some calories truly are better (or worse) than others.

Wrong Again

Despite its questionable values or benefits to our diets at all, sugar has largely escaped the public wrath of dieters and nutritionists alike. Instead, the main culprit of recent history has been presumed to be dietary fat.

In the 1940s, a physiology and nutrition researcher at the University of Minnesota, Dr. Ancel Keys, noticed the incredibly low incidence of heart disease in many European countries, particularly in areas such as Italy and Greece around the Mediterranean Sea. Meanwhile, in the United States, heart disease was becoming increasingly problematic, especially among well-to-do businessmen who, in theory, had the most access to good food and health care in the population.

Keys chalked up the differences in cardiovascular problems to diet: the Mediterranean diet consisted of lots of varied fruits and vegetables and lean fats, such as olive oil. The typical American diet, however, was very high in fat, especially animal fats. Keys hypothesized that saturated fat was the main culprit behind heart disease. He drew up a correlative study that measured the rate of saturated fat consumption with the rate of heart disease across seven countries; the results supported his hypothesis, and his presentation of evidence to the American government and public proved hugely influential, landing him on the cover of *TIME* magazine in January 1961.

Not everyone was convinced. Of all the countries in the world, Keys based his findings on only men in seven of them — the United States, Finland, the Netherlands, Italy, Yugoslavia, Greece, and Japan. Notably absent were countries and cultures whose traditional diets are high in animal fats like the American Inuit, for example, or the French. Had Keys included more countries, critics say, he might not have found such a strong correlation. Nevertheless, American nutritionists, including those of the USDA, began recommending that consumers reduce their intake of saturated fat in order to prevent heart disease. That was over fifty years ago; our fat consumption has since gone down, but our heart disease rates are higher than ever.

Meanwhile, in London, another physiologist/nutritionist, Dr. John Yudkin, pointed out an equally strong correlation between the incidence of heart disease by country with its people's rates of refined sugar consumption. Yudkin's 1972 book, *Pure, White, and Deadly*, argued that it was sugar, not fat, causing obesity, diabetes, and heart disease. While it earned high sales on both sides of the Atlantic, Yudkin's theory failed to have the same sweeping effect in the U.S. as Minnesota's own Ancel Keys' theory.

Between the 1950s and 1970s, butter and egg consumption dropped in the U.S. while the use of vegetable oils and sugars increased.[70] As Americans became increasingly conscious of their fat intake, food manufacturers rushed to meet the demand for low-fat products of all kinds, from yogurt and cheese to cookies and potato chips. Of course, once the fat was removed from many of these foods, the taste suffered; to keep a delicious appeal, the companies simply swapped in sugar for fat.

The results — or lack of them — say it all. Over one hundred years since we first started counting calories, and fifty years since we started trimming fat from our diets, Americans are more overweight than ever and increasingly at risk for heart disease.

Our diets and change in diet haven't worked. When we reexamine the old theories that a calorie is just a calorie and that fat begets fat, we begin to see why. And we begin to find our way toward solutions.

PART III:

Sweet Suffering

Sugar and Biological Disease

CHAPTER 7

Lost in the Supermarket

TO QUANTIFY THE PROBLEM of sugar in our diet, we'd want to first determine a baseline of how much we're eating. Good luck with that.

The simple awareness of sugar — how it floods our diets, shapes our culture, and affects our society — can turn a benign grocery store into a confusing maze. Sugar can hide in so many places because it comes in so many forms. When we think of "sugar," we tend only to imagine a mound of pure white crystals, but that's not how we usually encounter and consume it.

Let's take a walk through the average American supermarket. In the produce section, you'll find fruits, vegetables, tubers — things that are grown out of the ground or picked from a tree and delivered, mostly unaltered, to the store stands and shelves. There are no refined sugars here, but there are sugars.

They occur naturally, of course, in everything from apples and beets, from carrots to spinach. But when you pick up a beet in the produce section, you're also getting the fiber, water, vitamins, and minerals that make it up. Refined sugar, on the other hand, is a plant without all the other elements that make it a plant. With beet sugar, for example, every part of the beet except the sugar is removed and discarded to make pure white sugar.

When you eat fruits and vegetables in their whole form, the sugars don't count as refined or added. They're intrinsically a part of the food, and the food could not exist without them. So please, eat as many whole fruits and vegetables as you want!

Outside the grocery store's earthy produce section, though, sugars get trickier. Let's walk to the dairy section. Whether skim, whole, or 2%, any gallon of milk will show 12 grams of sugar per cup on its label. How can that be if there isn't anything in that gallon besides cow's milk itself?

The milk of all mammals, cows and humans alike, contains a kind of sugar called lactose. Lactose is a bigger sugar made up of two smaller sugars, glucose and galactose — an entirely different kind of sugar than the kind found in plants or in canisters at the coffee counter. The sugar we know and love — the pure white sugar — is called sucrose. Sucrose, like lactose, is a bigger sugar made up of two smaller sugars: glucose and fructose. Fruits and vegetables often contain sucrose, but they might also contain freestanding glucose or fructose.

So here's the basic summary of sugar's composition, which becomes important to know as we pinpoint how sugars affect us:

- Glucose is the baseline sugar. It appears in almost every living thing on earth. Foods that are starches, like potatoes and grains, consist of chains of glucose. Even though they're not sweet, they still contain sugar.
- Galactose is the milk sugar. When combined with glucose, it forms a larger sugar called lactose.
- Fructose is the "sweet sugar." When combined with glucose, it forms a larger sugar called sucrose.

A grape and an apple both contain sucrose. But they also contain varying amounts of glucose and fructose that float free and unattached from each other. Grapes contain more fructose, proportionally, than do most kinds of apples, which is why grapes taste sweeter than apples. Plain milk, however, only contains lactose.

The trouble is, all of these sugars are very different from each other and react in our bodies in different ways — but we still call all of them "sugar." If we turn our attention to the nutrition label on the chocolate milk down the aisle from the plain milk, this generalization becomes problematic. If a cup of chocolate milk contains 27 grams of sugar, what does that mean? Logically, we can deduce that if a cup of plain milk contains 12 grams of sugar in the form of lactose, then the chocolate milk also contains 12 grams of lactose. That leaves 15 grams of other sugars *added* to the product, probably in the form of sucrose or high-fructose corn syrup.

The key word is *probably*. With current nutrition labeling practices, we have no way of knowing. And the confusion only gets worse. Farther along down the dairy aisle, we might pick up some flavored yogurt — strawberry, let's say. The label of a six-ounce container says there are 28 grams of sugar inside. But what kind of sugars? To compare, we might search for a nearby plain yogurt of the same brand to see how many of those sugars are milk-sugar lactose: 13 grams. That leaves another 15 grams of sugar unaccounted for. We might read the first few ingredients: milk, sugar, strawberries. But how many of those 15 grams of non-milk sugars come from the strawberries, and how many from sucrose?

Not-So-Super Market

If this seems like an awful lot of work to uncover a simple answer, that's because it is. But as we'll see in the coming chapters, it matters whether your sugar comes from milk, strawberries, or sucrose. It matters whether it's whole or refined. It matters whether it's just a part of the food or if a manufacturer has added it. The less information we have detailing exactly how much and what kind of sugar we're eating, the more difficult it is to see how it all adds up in terms of our individual and societal health.

And still, we haven't even made it into the main aisles of the supermarket. It's obvious that the soda, cookie, and candy aisles will be filled with sugary snacks, but even here it's difficult to tell how much or what kind. Sugar hides under many names: sugar, sucrose, high-fructose corn syrup, evaporated cane juice, date syrup, fruit juice concentrate, turbinado, panocha, golden syrup, dextrose, Florida crystals, castor sugar, and more. They're all code names for the same thing: added refined sugars.

Not only might we be eating sugars without even recognizing its name on a label, but we can easily be deceived about how much sugar any given product really contains. A savvy, health-conscious consumer knows better than to buy a product that lists sugar as its first ingredient, since the law requires food manufacturers to list product ingredients on the nutrition label in order of weight. That jar of grape jam that reads "Ingredients: Sugar, Grapes" contains more added sugar than it does actual grapes.

But here, food manufacturers have found a loophole to outwit us: By using multiple types of sugar (in essence, using many names for a very similar substance), sugar no longer jumps out as the first ingredient. If we care that our grape jam contains more grapes than it does sugar, we look to see that grapes are listed as the first ingredient. But what does it mean if an ingredient list reads "Grapes, Sugar, High-Fructose Corn Syrup"? Yes, there are more grapes than sugar, and more grapes than high-fructose corn syrup, but if we were to add the amounts of sugar and high-fructose corn syrup together (which are, to the body, essentially the same thing), would they outweigh the number of grapes? Again, we don't know — and we can't know, given the information made available to us.

Food label literacy is vital to recognizing and realizing the swarm of sugars around us and learning how to avoid them. When we start meandering the aisles of the supermarket, reading labels on everything from salad dressing to crackers to canned soups and sauces, it becomes grossly apparent how much sugar there is in virtually every food product on the shelves.

The amount of addition, subtraction, decoding, close reading, and pure guesswork required to figure out just how much sugar a product contains makes it very difficult to track exactly how much we eat every day. It's easy for even the small, hidden sugars to add up to large amounts over the course of a day, a month, and years of consumption.

With supersize grocery stores and the dizzying array of products on every shelf, we like to think we have choices in how and what we eat. In reality, so much of our food is simply a clever variation of a similar theme, with sugar appearing in virtually all of it.

What does all that sugar actually do to our bodies? A look at the biology tells two shockingly different stories, depending on how we consume it.

CHAPTER 8

A Flood of Sugar

To most people, the word "sugar" simply means the sweet white granules that come in five-pound bags at the supermarket. But remember, what we know as table sugar — or its scientific name, sucrose — is actually made up of two simpler sugars, or saccharides: glucose and fructose. These, along with galactose (found only in mammal's milk), are the three primary sugars in the human diet.

Glucose is a carbohydrate, which simply means it contains a combination of carbon, hydrogen, and oxygen, and is the very life force of every living thing on earth. It is the product of photosynthesis in plants and is the easiest way for animals to convert food into fuel.

But *how* glucose gets into our blood streams makes all the difference. A sweet apple and a sweet candy bar are both packed with glucose, so it might seem like they'd be equally good energy sources. Biochemically, however, an apple and a candy bar do very different things to our bodies.

When you eat an apple, the fiber it contains acts like a casing around the glucose. Before the small intestine — where most digestion occurs — can absorb sugars or any other form of carbohydrate, it must first use digestive enzymes to break down layers of hard fiber that the body can't absorb. Only then can it access the calories inside and distribute them throughout the body for fuel. The result is a slow, more gradual rise in blood sugar levels, leading to a healthier rate of insulin release by the pancreas. Fiber slows down digestion and prolongs it so that a small, steady stream of energy can enter the body gradually and keep us energized for long periods of time. It's the fiber in food that makes us feel full, helping to trigger us to stop eating once we've received enough energy. (The hormone leptin plays a crucial role here as well; more on that later.) Fiber keeps us regulated, in more ways than one.

But when you eat a candy bar — or anything else with lots of refined sugar but little or no fiber — the calories become readily available. Without fiber, the small intestine absorbs them immediately and all at once instead of having to gradually work through fiber's shell. The result this time is a faster rise in our blood sugar level. We may get a rapid surge of energy from foods without fiber — including refined sugars, fruit juices, and even fiber-stripped grains like white bread and white rice — but because they're absorbed so quickly, the feeling of fullness doesn't last. Just as quickly as we eat, the energy passes through our bodies, which causes us to seek out more energy and more food, more times throughout the day.

The rapid absorption of refined sugars is the start of many health problems. It's very important to note that when we talk about "refined sugars" here, it doesn't just mean the kind you use for baking. It also includes commercial sweeteners of any kind, including honey, pure cane sugar, and high-fructose corn syrup alike. It also means fruit juices from concentrate and fruit juices pressed right before your eyes, because much of the fiber gets strained out in the juice-making process. It includes instant mashed potatoes and soft, fluffy white bread. It means any kind of carbohydrate that enters the body without the benefit of fiber — any food that has been deliberately stripped of its fiber content for ease, convenience or palatability. From the body's perspective, all of these look the same; they all look like sugar.

It's simple enough to pour a cup of crystal white sugar into your favorite cookie recipe. It'd be much harder to try to cram four sugar beets in there — which is how many plants it takes to produce a single cup of refined sugar. The beet is only 20% sugar; the rest is water, fiber, minerals and micronutrients. Consuming whole foods like fruits and vegetables helps prevent us from eating too much at once. To get to the sugars in a beet, we need to consume all the water and fiber along with it, which would leave us feeling very full and hydrated.

When we turn plants like beets, cane, corn, or agave into sugar, we leave the majority of the food behind, along with all of its vitamins, minerals, and macronutrients such as protein and fats. The same goes for fruit juices, no matter how fresh or pure. Why is it that it's so easy and quick to drink a glass of orange juice with breakfast, but to sit down and eat four oranges (the amount of fruit it takes to make that cup of juice) plus a regular meal would probably make us feel uncomfortably full? There's water in fruit juice, of course, but there's little or no fiber.

When we extract the sugar from our foods, we end up with a highly concentrated part removed from the whole. We've taken the part of the plant we like most — the sweetness — and isolated it from its larger parts so that we can consume more of it much more quickly. With technologies that weed out all the excess and provide us only the sugar, we're suddenly able to consume much, much more sugar at once than our bodies were ever meant to do.

Overload in the Liver

The stomach and intestines do most of the work required to break down our food, but in reality the digestive process — and the difference between that fibrous apple and nonfibrous candy bar — has only just begun. The process of metabolism is how the food we eat becomes the energy we use, but the body metabolizes different foods in different ways.

Glucose can be used by any cell in the body that needs some fuel, which is why it's generally considered the body's preferred source of energy. Glucose transports itself through the bloodstream as it waits for a cell in need of its energies. Our "blood sugar" level should more accurately be called a "blood glucose" level, since it's a measure of only the amounts of glucose — not fructose or galactose — in the blood at any given time. Glucose levels in the blood are closely monitored by the hormone insulin, which directs glucose energy to the places it's most needed; more glucose in the blood requires more insulin to take charge and direct it appropriately. Insulin, in turn, triggers another hormone, leptin, which produces both physical and mental cues that make us stop eating. Once insulin has ensured that all cells have received the appropriate amount of glucose, it cues leptin to make us feel full so we'll stop eating. That prevents an overload of glucose from flooding the body.

At the same time, glucose can also be taken up by the liver and converted into glycogen, which act as reserves for times when available food energy is low. Between meals, if our cells require more energy, the liver will emit just enough glucose into the bloodstream to keep us active and alert.

Other foods undergo a different metabolic process: Fats, proteins, and the sugar fructose all must be processed by the liver first before they can be used as energy by the cells. *This is a crucial difference.* Even though fructose is a carbohydrate, too, it doesn't get metabolized the same way glucose does. Fructose is metabolized in the same way as a fat or protein — through the liver. Curiously, it seems to be the only type of carbohydrate to do so.

Fructose, in many ways, is still a mysterious molecule. Whereas glucose provides instant energy, and fats and proteins help build and maintain important cellular structures, fructose doesn't seem to serve any biological purpose. So what is it doing in our foods?

In nature — that is, in anything that grows out of the ground as opposed to processed foods — fructose is never found alone. It is always paired with glucose; not necessarily bound together, as in table sugar, but at least co-existent. There is no food that contains only fructose and no glucose.

Evolutionarily, this seems to make sense: fructose is the sweet part of sugar, the part that makes our food taste so good. It makes fruits attractive and delicious. But, importantly, those fruits also contain high amounts of glucose (to give us energy) and fiber (which helps make us feel full). Fructose is the showpiece sugar; it doesn't necessarily lend a hand in digestion or metabolism, but it's what motivates us to eat food in the first place. Our hunter-gatherer ancestors who were fortunate enough to find an ample source of fructose — a patch of ripe berries, for instance — would have eaten as much of the sweet, delicious fruit as possible, and their bodies would have saved the excess stores of energy from glucose for later.

In our society, of course, it's much easier to find fructose. We no longer have to scrounge for wild berries — or even wait for them to be in season; we can simply pick them up at the store. We don't even have to eat whole fruits in order to get a satisfactory dose of fructose. We can get it in conveniently processed and refined candies, fruit juices, and baked goods packed with sucrose. Needless to say, we're consuming far more fructose than our ancestors ever did — or, indeed, than our biological evolution prepared us to have. (We eat an average of 70 pounds a year, far more than a century ago). Our bodies are not equipped to handle all of the fructose that's so readily accessible.

When we eat refined sugars, as in a candy bar with no fiber, blood glucose levels spike incredibly high and incredibly quickly. The insulin secreted needs to find a way to deal with the sudden flood of glucose in the bloodstream, and quickly. Most of it gets shipped to the liver as excess to be converted to glycogen. Meanwhile, the liver is also trying to process and metabolize the candy bar's fructose. With refined-sugar foods that contain both glucose and fructose — in essence, all sweeteners — the liver is inundated with excess glucose from the blood at the exact same time it's trying to process fructose. High amounts of refined sugars end up slamming the liver with double duty.

It doesn't matter what kind of sugar it is. White, brown, raw, turbinado — those are all sucrose, which is considered the benchmark for sweetness because it always contains an equal proportion of glucose and fructose. Other sweeteners might bear different profiles — high-fructose corn syrup, as we stated earlier, contains roughly 55% fructose and 45% glucose, although the mixture can vary. But again: biochemically, they are all pretty much the same to our bodies, no matter what we call them.

If the body is subjected to these spikes of refined sugar repeatedly and regularly — a soda or sports drink habit, for example, or a constant intake of fiber-less foods — it will come to expect and anticipate the high sugar load.

Our bodies have an amazing capacity to adapt to their surroundings — but in this case, that's not doing us any favors.

If our blood glucose levels spike unusually high every time we eat, the body will react by keeping some extra insulin on hand at all times, to be prepared for these onslaughts of glucose. That means higher baseline levels of insulin that are at the ready in the bloodstream at all times. The trouble is, insulin only acts once we reach a certain level of glucose concentration. When the baseline insulin level stays higher, we need equally higher amounts of glucose to use up the right amount of energy and then signal the leptin hormone to start making us feel full. If we don't feel full right away, we tend to eat more, pushing more glucose into our blood than we need, triggering more insulin to go out and manage it. The body starts to think it needs *more* insulin at the ready for every time we eat, and then *that* level is established as the new insulin baseline, requiring *more* glucose to kick it into action.

As you can see, too much refined sugar creates a vicious cycle: we require greater and greater amounts of food (specifically carbohydrates) just to feel satiated; meanwhile, those foods are often making the problem worse. Our system, in a way, becomes dependent on those high surges of refined carbohydrates because it's what the body has come to know and expect. Even with attempts to eat healthily, we might be left feeling unfulfilled or hungry without that little extra spike of sugar that really kicks our hormones into gear. It's not that there's not enough insulin; the body has simply become unresponsive to it.

This is not a change that happens overnight. One candy bar won't send your metabolic hormones into an irrevocable downward spiral. It's the habitual pattern of consumption over weeks, months, and years that gradually changes the way the body responds. These are the long-term side effects of excess sugar consumption, and they can be extremely difficult to reverse or overcome.

Domino Effect

Once insulin — the key regulator of our metabolism — gets thrown off by sugars, other systems begin to fail to respond properly, too. We may gain weight as the body looks for new ways to store excess glucose. We may lose the ability to regulate our blood sugar levels completely, a condition known as type 2 diabetes. These two factors establish particularly worrisome precedents for more dangerous conditions down the road: high blood pressure, high cholesterol, and, eventually, heart disease.

A person with chronically high levels of insulin whose body fails to respond to it in normal ways is deemed "insulin resistant." Insulin resistance is the underlying factor in a host of maladies, including obesity, type 2 diabetes, hypertension, elevated triglycerides, and low protective (HDL) cholesterol. Very often, all five of these risk factors occur simultaneously. Having one is a strong predictor of developing another, because they all trace back to the malfunction of insulin. And if you have three of the five, you qualify for a larger condition that's known as *metabolic syndrome*, and the consequences could be severe.

Insulin itself isn't the problem with metabolic syndrome; it's the rest of the body's failure to respond to its messages. Essentially, our metabolic systems become desensitized to perpetually high levels of insulin and stop paying attention to the usual trigger cues. The cells stop absorbing energy properly. Leptin doesn't fire like it should, and so we never feel full. The liver won't keep excess sugars on hand for energy but instead will send them off to be stored as fat that accumulates first on our stomach and thighs, and then eventually around the vital organs and arterial walls, which can be extremely dangerous to our physical health.

While the risk factors of metabolic syndrome aren't always deadly in and of themselves, they serve as an extremely high predictor of America's number one killer: heart disease. Though metabolic syndrome is technically defined as the presence of three or more of the risk factors included in its symptoms, nearly half of all adult Americans exhibit signs of at least one, which in turn elevates the risk for the development of others. Thirty-four percent of

Americans *already* have three or more and are considered extremely at-risk for heart disease. Metabolic syndrome doubles the chances of developing atherosclerosis — the hardening of the artery walls most commonly associated with heart attack or heart failure.[71]

A Way Out?

Yet underlying all this is good news. Nearly every cause of metabolic syndrome comes down to life choices. While genetics do play some role in the risk of heart disease, up to 90% of the odds of developing it are determined by diet and lifestyle.[72] It's a remarkable fact: the vast majority of all cases of heart disease are preventable.

Over the past fifty years, our medical technologies, understandings, and methods of treating heart disease and its precursory elements have grown exponentially. Yet our rates of death by heart disease have skyrocketed.

Nearly one in three deaths in the United States can be attributed to cardiovascular (heart) disease. One out of every six dollars spent on health care in our country goes directly toward treating heart disease or metabolic syndrome — that's $444 billion every year, more than a dollar every second of every minute of every day. If current rates and patterns continue, the costs and incidences of heart disease alike are projected to triple by as early as 2030.[73] I can't stress enough that this is a *preventable* disease, a preventable expense, and a preventable death. Treatments are expensive; prevention shouldn't have to be.

Heart disease doesn't simply fall randomly from the sky; it's the result of years of habits that gradually take a toll on our bodies. But we understand better now than ever before how and why heart disease develops over the course of a lifetime, why metabolic syndrome is such a strong predictive factor of heart disease, and the potential role that sugar plays in bringing about metabolic syndrome. The true culprit has been staring us right in the face all these years.

It's absolutely vital to recognize that the long flow of chain reactions in our bodies that wind up producing such terrible diseases all start with the simple act of eating. Ultimately, we have to understand the consequences of our actions, starting with our forks.

People have known — or at least suspected — for centuries that sugar can lead to some awful side effects, whether it's the Queen's rotten black teeth or the old "pissing evil," diabetes. Current science helps us understand why, not just as we eat during a meal, but as we eat over the course of a lifetime.

What's the Damage?

Let's tackle a graph demonstrating how excess sugar/carb consumption leads to all the diseases associated with metabolic syndrome. The criteria for metabolic syndrome for which 1/3 of Americans suffer are:

(1)   Waist circumference, the criteria that correlates the most with subsequent disease: For men, greater than 40 inch waist circumference; for women, greater than 35 inches.
(2) Elevated fasting blood glucose (above 105)
(3) Elevated triglycerides (above 150)
(4) Elevated blood pressure (above 140/90)
(5) Reduced "good" HDL level (for men, less than 35; women, less than 40)

Though the graph looks complicated, it is easy to follow if you read the numbered explanation that corresponds to the appropriate portion of the graph. Every disease presented results from excess sugar consumption (especially fructose).

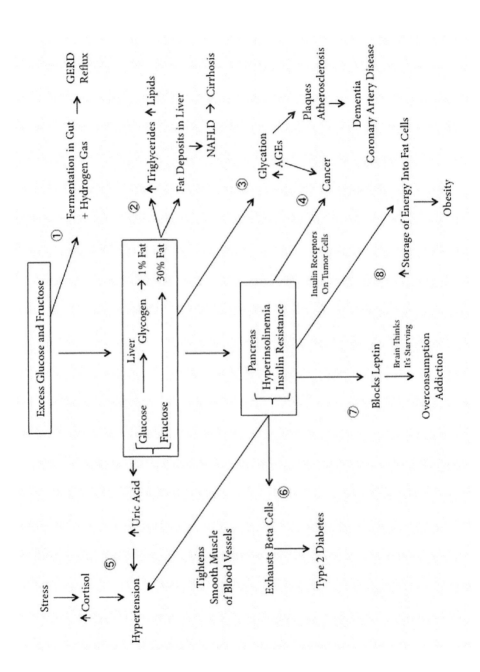

(1) There's some early evidence suggesting refined carbohydrates, like sugars, might aggravate acid reflux and GERD, since excess carbohydrate load leads to fermentation in the gut and a resultant increase in hydrogen gas production that can drive acidic stomach contents backwards through the lower esophageal sphincter. However, these studies were based on a very limited sample size and need to be more fully explored.[74, 75]

(2) Excess sugar is processed in the liver. Glucose is converted to glycogen for future use; only 1% is converted to fat. Fructose is another story. It is only metabolized in the liver; 30% is converted into fat! Over time, the fatty deposits in the liver lead to nonalcoholic fatty liver disease (NAFLD) and ultimately cirrhosis of the liver. The fat produced by fructose metabolism also increases triglycerides, leading to hyperlipidemia.

(3) Excess sugar attaches to fat and protein, distorting their shape and rendering them dysfunctional. This glycation process leads to the formation of advanced glycogen end products (AGEs), which clump together. The resulting plaques lead to blockages in the brain and arteries ultimately causing strokes, dementia, and myocardial infarction.

(4) Cancer can result both from the accumulation of AGEs and from the incorporation of excess glucose into the tumor cell (via insulin receptors) which leads to tumor growth.

(5) Hypertension results from two unique pathways. First, excess fructose is metabolized to uric acid, which increases blood pressure — and causes gout. Secondly, hyperinsulinemia causes the smooth muscle surrounding blood vessels to constrict, resulting in high blood pressure.

(6) Prolonged exposure to excess sugar makes the beta cells in the pancreas work overtime to produce the insulin needed to maintain a normal blood glucose level. Eventually the pancreas can't keep up with demand and it begins to fatigue, leading to type 2 diabetes and the need for metformin or insulin treatment. Chronic elevations in insulin lead to insulin resistance.

(7) Hyperinsulinemia and insulin resistance influence the biomedical pathways that result in overconsumption and addiction.

(8) Hyperinsulinemia perpetually drives fat into cells, locks it there, and throws away the key, resulting in obesity.

This is a lot of information to take in all at once. Let's examine each of these effects in detail, and we'll begin to see how this map of sugar-related problems really plays out in the body.

CHAPTER 9

No Symptoms, Real Problem

YOU MIGHT HAVE THE BEGINNINGS of diabetes without even knowing it. It used to be a rare disease, but by 2020, it's projected that more than half of Americans will be diabetic or pre-diabetic. In 2014, it was estimated that as many as 35% of Americans were pre-diabetic, meaning they exhibited abnormally high blood sugar levels (or blood glucose levels, as I prefer to call it) without any of the outward symptoms of diabetes such as excessive thirst, increased urination, vision trouble, or dry skin. Early intervention is key in preventing the onset of full-blown type 2 diabetes, but pre-sufferers might not even be aware that they're already on their way.

Remember that when we talk about "blood sugar" levels, we're really only measuring the amount of glucose in the blood. So while there's a certain amount of various sugars coursing through our bloodstream at all times, we only register the amount of glucose — not fructose, not galactose — on our readings.

A healthy blood glucose concentration is typically considered less than 100 milligrams of sugar per deciliter of blood (mg/dL), which comes out to about five grams of glucose throughout the body's five or so liters of blood at any given time. Our hormones, especially insulin, run a tight ship on glucose levels, monitoring it and keeping it stable enough throughout the day to give us energy between meals and even during extended fasts. When there's a surge of available glucose, such as after eating, insulin quickly works to distribute energy from glucose to any and all cells as needed and then suppresses the amount of glucose circulating in the blood so that nothing goes to waste.

Glucose levels naturally rise and fall throughout the day as we consume and expend energy but, ideally, that 100mg/dL mark remains the target balance. Too little blood sugar and we may feel faint, shaky, and hungry — a problem usually fixed simply by eating something. Too *much* blood sugar is a much more difficult problem to solve.

The body's first line of defense against high blood-glucose concentrations is insulin, which directs glucose to be stored as fat for later use. As I described in the last chapter, the body will produce more insulin to deal with repeated surges of high glucose, which can lead to insulin resistance. This is the pre-diabetes stage. But even this cycle has its breaking point. In extreme cases, the body will flush out excess glucose through urinary excretion. This is when pre-diabetes becomes full-blown diabetes, and this is why diabetics have sweet-smelling urine: it's actually full of sugar.

Passing glucose through urine is not healthy for the body, especially the kidneys. It puts an enormous strain on their filtering capabilities, and over time can exhaust their ability to function. The kidneys will get so tired, they eventually fatigue and stop working entirely. Kidney failure is what eventually killed most people in the era before we understood the mechanics of type 2 diabetes. That's why it truly is the pissing evil.

An excessive amount of sweet-smelling urine is one of the hallmark symptoms of diabetes, but clinically, we define it as a chronic blood glucose level above 126mg/dL. Any level that's consistently over 100mg/dL, though, indicates a problem in the relationship between glucose and insulin and might be a cause for concern.

There's a Difference

Some people — fewer than one out of every 500 in the U.S. — lose the ability to produce insulin at all at a very young age. The telltale signs of diabetes — excess thirst, hunger, frequent urination, and weight loss — emerge early in childhood, as the body is unable to control its blood glucose levels except through kidney excretion. This is type 1 diabetes, an autoimmune disorder, and unlike type 2, it's defined by the body's inability to produce insulin, rather than type 2's inability to react even to high amounts of insulin. Though we still don't understand what triggers the sudden absence of insulin hormones, most type 1 cases are now managed effectively through injections of synthetic insulin into the bloodstream.

Other people — currently, about 1 in 10 in the United States — develop diabetes in spite of a rather abundant ability to produce insulin for most of their lives. Type 2 diabetes arises from the rest of the body's refusal to acknowledge insulin's signals. Normally, when large amounts of glucose enter the bloodstream, insulin triggers the cells to absorb energy. But as we've said, a chronically high level of insulin stemming from high glucose intake causes the body to develop an immunity to insulin. Other insulin-triggered hormones, like the appetite-suppressing leptin, also stop being effective. It's almost as if insulin is caught in a "hormone who cried wolf" situation; the warning signals of high blood glucose are fired, but the rest of the body has learned to ignore any false signs of potential danger. Eventually, insulin-producing cells may weaken and lose their ability to produce sufficient insulin to control blood sugar levels, just like what happens to kids with type 1 diabetes.

Type 2 used to be called "adult-onset" diabetes, but increasingly, that's becoming a misnomer as more and more teenagers and even young kids are turning up with insulin resistance instead of insulin deficiency. Type 2 diabetes is catastrophically on the rise, and it's this condition we need to worry about because we know it's related to dietary choices and sugar. In short, we know it's preventable.

Fifty years ago, less than 1% of the American population had diabetes of any kind, either autoimmune (type 1) or metabolic (type 2). Today, an estimated 13% of Americans over the age of 20 have diabetes, though many go undiagnosed. The vast majority of that increase is due to type 2 cases — and those numbers are expected to rise by a frightening 160% before 2050.[76, 77]

Untreated diabetes impairs glucose absorption throughout the body, which can lead to complications like vision loss, nerve damage and poor circulation that may lead to lower-body ulcers, kidney failure, increased risk of stroke and heart disease, or the need for limb amputations. Diabetes — and its accompanying problems — is the seventh leading cause of death in the U.S. today, directly causing 70,000 fatalities every year, though cardiovascular disease remains the leading cause of death among diabetics. The life expectancy of people with type 2 diabetes is a full ten years shorter, and they carry twice the risk of death as their non-diabetic peers at any age.

Of all the conditions of metabolic syndrome, diabetes is most inextricably linked with refined sugar consumption. Women who drink just one sweetened beverage per day, like fruit juice or soda, have an 83% greater chance of developing type 2 diabetes in their lifetimes than women who consume one or fewer sugary drink per month; and every additional drink ups the chances by another 25%.[78]

Diabetics have to carefully monitor their consumption of glucose, but that's not the only sugar causing problems.

The Lifelong Habit

Fructose, the other part of sugars and syrups, is different. It has no effect on blood glucose levels, which also means it has no direct effect on insulin, leptin, or other blood sugar-related hormones. As I've mentioned, and as we'll discuss in more depth in later chapters, fructose can only be metabolized by the liver. It's processed similarly to a lipid or protein in the liver, first being converted into triglycerides (clumps of lipids, or basically fat) and then transported through the bloodstream via clumps of fat and cholesterol known as lipoproteins. Fructose seems to be the only carbohydrate to get this unique kind of treatment, which can quickly become problematic for the heart and the vascular system.

Initially, fructose was heralded as a safe sweetener alternative for diabetics since it doesn't affect blood glucose levels. Fructose-only sweeteners were chemically and commercially developed, and agave nectar, a syrupy sweetener made from desert plants and containing a naturally high percentage of fructose, had a sudden heyday among TV-friendly doctors and health nuts. But with more recent research, it appears the opposite is true about fructose.

Lab studies demonstrate that animals fed only fructose were *more* likely to develop insulin resistance than animals fed only glucose, and were also at greater risk for other factors of metabolic syndrome, including abdominal obesity, high blood pressure and triglycerides, and fatty liver disease.[79]

Small amounts of fructose in the diet, especially when derived from whole fruits, may actually be beneficial in glucose control, however, there seems to be a threshold for toxicity for fructose, just as there is for alcohol and other substances, when we consume too much of it. As our consumption of refined sugars has risen over the years, so has our consumption of fructose: if the average American consumes 120 grams of refined sugar every day (less than 100 pounds per year, a conservative estimate), 60 grams or more of those sugars are fructose. You would have to eat roughly nine apples, or two pounds of cherries, or 22 bananas in one day to obtain that much fructose in your diet through fruits alone — but it only takes two and a half cans of Coke.

How much fructose is too much? Unfortunately, the answer isn't entirely clear. It's extremely difficult, if not downright impossible and unethical, to conduct controlled, long-term human experiments on matters of diet and nutrition, especially for something as ubiquitous as sugar. As with alcohol or tobacco, the detrimental health effects of fructose abuse can take years or even decades to emerge. It's not the one soda — or the one beer, or the one cigarette — that creates an immediate problem; it's the lifelong habit.

At the same time, there's no such thing as too *little* fructose: people born with hereditary fructose intolerance, an inability to process fructose sugars, are able to lead completely normal and healthy lives as long as they avoid that kind of sugar. There's no danger in reducing our fructose consumption — but there are very clear toxic consequences for taking in too much.

Telltale Statistics

Looking at the historical patterns of disease and sugar consumption, a few trends jump out immediately. Rates for obesity, diabetes, and heart disease have all nearly doubled in the United States since the late 1980s. Assuming it can take up to twenty years for a sugar-eating habit to manifest as a health problem — as is usually the case with smoking and lung cancer, for example — the spike in metabolic disease correlates perfectly with the spike in American sugar consumption in the late 1960s and early 1970s, after the introduction of high-fructose corn syrup in the commercial sweetener market. Per-capita consumption of caloric sweeteners (table sugar, HFCS, honey, etc.) first topped 120 pounds per person per year in 1971. Today, we're approaching roughly 160 pounds annually.

It's not one or the other — fructose or glucose — that's the main culprit; it's the combination of the two. Glucose directly disturbs insulin while fructose disrupts liver metabolism, and together the problems compound into a perfect storm for the development of not only type 2 diabetes but also an increased risk for all of the other risk factors of metabolic syndrome: obesity, low protective (HDL) cholesterol, hypertension, high triglycerides, and ultimately atherosclerosis and heart disease.

Yet diabetes doesn't always come first; the presence of any one condition of metabolic syndrome increases the chances of developing type 2 diabetes. This suggests that no one condition causes the other but, instead, they share a common underlying link: namely, glucose-fructose (i.e., refined sugar and sweetener) consumption.

Conventional wisdom has long blamed dietary fat — not sugar— as a primary cause of heart disease. Although there's an extraordinarily high incidence of heart disease in people with type 2 diabetes, they're usually treated as separate issues; one caused by fat, the other by sugar, but both involving poor diet and exercise habits. But the clear links between sugar and diabetes, and the links between diabetes and heart disease, mean we need to rethink these assumptions. Dietary fat consumption cannot explain all the symptoms of metabolic syndrome, but sugar can. Refined sugar is most likely the true instigator of metabolic disease, as well as its fatal bedmates: cardiac arrest and stroke.

In the medical professions and as a popular society at large, our attempts to solve and prevent heart disease by reducing dietary fat have produced pitifully few results. No matter how good our intentions are, we've simply been barking up the wrong tree.

What we know about diabetes can lead us to answers about other diseases, but only if we take the time to connect the dots. Like other conditions of metabolic syndrome, diabetes is preventable 9 times out of 10 through simple healthy lifestyle choices. Yet cases in the United States and around the world continue to soar. At continuing rates, nearly 600 million people worldwide will be living with diabetes by 2035. Rates are especially high in populations where traditional diets are being increasingly replaced with American-style convenience diets high in sugars from soft drinks and prepared foods; while the rate of diabetes in the U.S. is appalling as it is, eighty percent of all diabetes cases around the world occur in low- to middle-income countries, not our own.[80]

The real costs of diabetes in the United States are tremendous. Medical bills for someone with diabetes average $13,700 a year, more than twice that for someone without diabetes.[81] In 2012, between treatments and the economic productivity lost because of sick or absent workers, diabetes cost the nation $245 billion — a 41% increase over the previous five years. We owe it to our personal health, both physically and financially, to take the real prevention of diabetes seriously — especially knowing that where one disease lurks, the rest of the related metabolic syndrome diseases are likely to follow.

CHAPTER 10

Obesity

T HERE'S NO ARGUING THAT AMERICA is the most obese country in the world. But there's plenty of debate about why. It's a riddle we haven't been able to solve for thirty years or more, no matter the latest fad diet, workout craze, or superfood on the market. The American Medical Association (AMA), back in 1999, officially described rates of obesity in the United States as having reached epidemic proportions, noting how "rarely do chronic conditions such as obesity spread with the speed and dispersion characteristic of a communicable disease epidemic." The AMA was so alarmed and serious about the subject that they devoted an entire issue of the *Journal* to it.[82]

Their concern was justified: prevalence of obesity had taken a sharp upturn in less than a decade, from 12% of the population in 1991 to 18% in 1998. Despite continual research and awareness, that escalating trend hasn't changed. Today, nearly 33% of American adults are obese, and another 33% are overweight.

The clinical difference between being overweight and obese is defined using the Body Mass Index (BMI) height-to-weight ratio. To calculate your BMI, first multiply your weight in pounds by a conversion factor of 703, and then divide by your height (in inches) squared. So, for example, a five-foot-nine-inch person weighing 150 pounds would have a BMI of ﹍ within the healthy range. A BMI ratio over 25 is considered overw﹍ of 30 or more is considered obese. The formula, as everyone will ack﹍ isn't perfect because it doesn't directly measure body fat; a body buil﹍ instance, will likely have a very high weight-to-height ratio becau﹍ muscles, not fat — but in general, the BMI is a useful tool in gauging healtl﹍ a glance, even if no two bodies are alike.

There's nothing wrong with being overweight or obese in and of itself; it's the health risks that correlate highly with excess weight that are the issue. Even so, many people might be surprised to learn that obesity is not a prescription or even a necessary precursor for metabolic disease: approximately 30% of clinically obese people have none of the risk factors associated with metabolic syndrome. And as many as 40% of people in the normal-weight range actually have risk factors for metabolic syndrome.

The obesity epidemic remains such a hot-button issue in American society because excess weight is so highly linked with the other diseases of metabolic syndrome — and because it's the most outwardly visible symptom of possibly ill health (but again, only *possibly*). You don't necessarily have to go to the doctor to find out if you're overweight, the way you might have to in order to check your blood glucose levels or blood pressure. Appearances aside, the fact is that obesity and even being moderately overweight is associated with three to four times the risk for developing type 2 diabetes, as well as a greater risk for hypertension, high cholesterol, heart disease, and the overall chance of morbidity stemming from any one of these illnesses.[83]

Yet in many cases of obesity, even a 5% reduction in body mass can prevent, delay, or even reverse symptoms and diseases of metabolic syndrome.

Pick Your Poison

So where does obesity come from? Why and how do we get fat? That is the million-dollar question. If we had a clear, simple answer, we most likely wouldn't be in this mess. The typical American diet — full of pre-packaged foods and prepared meals, salty snacks, sweets, fatty meat, refined carbohydrates, and fast food—has no shortage of suspects. One out of every seven meals in the U.S. comes from a restaurant — and a whopping three-quarters of those from a fast food restaurant, where portions tend to be larger and the food itself much higher in fat, salt, and sugar than what most people would prepare at home. Compared to USDA recommendations, most Americans' diets are lacking in fruits, vegetables, and whole grains, while excessive in fat, salt, and sugar. Somehow I'm guessing you're not surprised.

Since the 1970s, most of the attention in the obesity wars has focused on fat. This view has been constantly propagated and reinforced by the government via its *Dietary Guidelines* published every five years, advising adults to limit fat intake to 30% or less of daily calories. The number of Americans observing a low-saturated fat diet (defined as less than 10% of daily calories) has increased from 25% of the population in the late 1970s to 42% today, but this has done nothing to reduce the upward trends of obesity and heart disease.

Consumption of refined sugars, on the other hand, has clearly risen. The average modern teenager consumes 17% of daily total calories in the form of added sugars (meaning at least 50% of the teenage population consumes even more). Teen and childhood rates of obesity, like that of the general population, have also swelled at alarming rates, from about 5% of all children in 1976 to 25% today. Of the 442 sugar calories teen boys consume on average every day, a full 273 (well over half) come just from beverages such as soda, fruit juice, and sports drinks.[84]

With so many variables — including levels of physical activity and genetics — it's impossible to lay complete blame for the obesity epidemic on one single food or commodity. But soft drinks might be a good place to start. For every soda consumed, the odds of developing obesity increase by 60%.[85] Caloric intake from sugar-sweetened drinks has more than doubled in the past fifty years; at an average 7.1% of total daily caloric consumption, beverages contribute more calories than any other single foodstuff in our diets. If the entire American population were to eliminate *only* sugar-sweetened carbonated sodas, we'd reduce our per capita sugar consumption by 39 pounds every year. Without soda, we might be consuming less sugar than what was strictly rationed out by the government during World War II.

Soft drinks and fruit juices, which are all essentially different variations on the sugar-water cocktail, are a potent example of how sugars act in the body to promote fat buildup. Glucose-fructose sweeteners, like table sugar, high-fructose corn syrup, fruit sugar, evaporated cane juice, etc., are a tag-team force that encourage the production of bodily fats in two ways: through insulin resistance in the blood and lipogenesis (conversion into fatty acids) in the liver.

Remember, glucose in the bloodstream normally stimulates the secretion of the hormone insulin, which in turn triggers the hormone leptin to help produce feelings of fullness after we eat. But with repeated surges of high glucose, as happens with sugars, soft drinks, and fruit juices, insulin levels can be thrown off balance, leading to the same type of insulin resistance characteristic of type 2 diabetes (and to diabetes itself).

Just as insulin adapts to persistently high levels of blood glucose, the appetite-suppressing hormone leptin adapts to persistently high levels of insulin. It takes higher and higher amounts of glucose to fire the signals that tell us we're full and should stop eating, which can make people eat more than they need for simple energy purposes.

With dysfunctional insulin and leptin, overeating — and, with it, weight gain and obesity — becomes a vicious cycle. The more excess energy consumed, the more the body comes to expect that same energy intake all the time. That's part of the reason why it can be so hard to lose weight, yet so easy to put it back on. Our bodies are happy to adapt for us, but once they do, it can be difficult to reverse the change.

Overconsumption

This next section choreographs how chronic overconsumption of sugar (especially fructose) leads to limitless appetite, addiction, and all the diseases associated with metabolic syndrome. Don't panic, the information will be summarized and simplified for those who don't wish to relive college. For those who are gluttons (sorry) for punishment, the accompanying graphs are worth understanding. Much of the information that follows is derived from Robert Lustig's work on sugar metabolism. He is the modern-day guru on the harmful effects of sugar consumption and I owe a great deal of my understanding to his efforts.[86]

The most important takeaways from the following pages are:

(1) Chronic overconsumption of sugar leads to hyperinsulinemia and subsequent insulin resistance.
(2) Fat cells produce leptin (the "I'm full and satisfied" hormone). Too much leptin leads to leptin resistance.
(3) Insulin blocks leptin.
(4) Limitless appetite, addiction, and the diseases associated with metabolic syndrome are all secondary to biochemical processes that we can't override.
(5) No one chooses to be obese or metabolically sick.

Healthy Appetite	Unhealthy Appetite
Consume Food	Consume Food
⬇	⬇
Normal Insulin	Excessive Insulin
⬇	✖
Leptin	Leptin
⬇	⬇
Hypothalamus (VMH)	Hypothalamus (VMH)
⬇	⬇
Not Hungry / Burn Energy	Hungry / Store Energy
⬇	⬇
Promotes Energy Expenditure and Fat Loss	Promotes Storage Of Fat and Energy (Increased Appetite)
	⬇
	OVERCONSUMPTION

First, I must say that these graphs are a toned down, *simplistic overview* of a **very** complex biological system. Second, if you are *leptin resistant* then the same flow occurs. Leptin resistance is secondary to both the overconsumption of sugar (especially fructose) and from being obese since obese people have more fat cells and, thus, produce more leptin. That being said, from this diagram, one can see that part of our brain called the Ventromedial Hypothalamus (VMH) controls energy storage vs. expenditure. Leptin, discovered in 1994, is a hormone produced from fat cells that signals to the VMH that we are full and that we have enough energy.[87]

In a healthy appetite pathway, the hypothalamus is stimulated by leptin and gives the signal that one is not hungry, thus it is time to burn the energy that was just consumed. This promotion of energy expenditure can lead to fat loss.

But what happens when insulin fails to trigger leptin or when a person becomes leptin resistant? The whole process goes in reverse and the pathway effectively produces the opposite signal: one is hungry, and it's time to store energy. This leads to increased appetite instead of the typical "I'm full" feeling. As such, the process promotes overconsumption and, thus, weight gain.

In response, the pancreas produces even more insulin, which shunts energy nonstop into the fat cells. It essentially locks the door of the fat cell and throws away the key. You *cannot* lose weight when hyperinsulinemia exists (and we make twice the amount of insulin we did 30 years ago) and when leptin is blocked. Obese people are essentially leptin resistant.

Again, no one chooses to be obese or lethargic. Insulin excess (insulin resistance) and the resulting blocking of leptin (leptin resistance) are a one-two punch that makes it virtually impossible to curb our addictive and consumptive behaviors.

Fructose: A Visceral Problem (And Solution)

While the glucose half of sugars wreaks havoc on the balance of our digestive hormones, the fructose half is being churned into fat by the liver through a process known as *de novo lipogenesis*. It's very similar to how alcohol is processed; excess carbohydrates from beer, wine or liquor — none of which provide ample energy sources for the body — are turned into fat, creating the "beer gut" phenomenon. A sugar gut is made the same way.

De novo lipogenesis is tough work for the liver, and the heavy strain over long periods of time can lead to an accumulation of fat on the liver itself, an undesirable condition known as fatty liver disease. Fatty liver disease can lead in turn to cirrhosis and even liver failure, both long-known consequences of alcoholism, and consequences of sugar-ism, too. Previously, fatty liver disease and cirrhosis were almost exclusively seen in alcoholics (at least ninety percent of alcohol abusers will develop fatty liver disease in their lifetimes). But increasingly since the 1980s, more and more cases of fatty liver disease are cropping up in patients who consume little or no alcohol, and even in young children.

A staggering 30% of the U.S. population now has fatty liver disease, nearly on par with rates of obesity and cardiovascular disease, and at least 70% of the people with non-alcoholic fatty liver disease (NAFLD) exhibit other facets of metabolic syndrome.[88] The only clinical difference between alcoholic fatty liver disease and the non-alcoholic kind is the source of the fat itself; since fructose metabolizes in the liver so similarly to alcohol, refined sugars are prime suspects in the recent prevalence of NAFLD. Independent of any other symptoms of metabolic syndrome, soft drink consumption is the single largest predictor of NAFLD. Sufferers are sometimes known to consume five times as many soft drinks as healthy individuals.[89]

Once the liver has converted fructose into fatty lipids, this fat has to either get used up in energy expenditure or stored somewhere for later. Lipids made from fructose tend to hang out in our abdominal (or visceral) fat, where they're easily accessed during periods of starvation or rapid energy expenditure such as exercise.

One of the reasons we crave sweets so much may be precisely for fructose's fat-inducing properties: during times of food scarcity, visceral fat would have safeguarded our ancestors from famine. Obviously, our current undiluted access to fructose produces more visceral fat than is good for us. Abdominal waist circumference and waist-to-hip ratios are two of the highest predictors of overall health — much more so than fat on the legs, butt, or arms, which can actually be indicators of good health. But too much visceral fat, on the other hand, can decrease life expectancy by as much as fifteen years.[90]

On the bright side, when weight loss does start to kick in, visceral fat is usually the first to go. But obesity remains a costly epidemic for the United States, where annual health care spending on issues of weight ($190 billion) now exceeds those caused by smoking. Average medical bills for obese men are $1,152 more per year than for non-obese, while the gap exceeds $3,600 for obese versus non-obese women.

Costs extend beyond just doctor's office visits. Our expanding waistlines demand bigger hospital beds, bigger transportation seating, even bigger coffins. The extra weight we carry around in our cars contributes to an estimated one billion gallons of extra gasoline use every year.[91] The non-obese also bear the brunt of costs in the form of higher health insurance premiums and lost productivity in the workplace, where obesity-related illnesses, doctor's visits, and "presenteeism" — the inability to perform at maximum capacity due to health issues — result in $506 of lost productivity per obese worker per year.[92]

By reducing or even eliminating refined sugars from our diet, we have little to lose and a lot to gain (or, from a weight perspective, we might say it the other way around). It's not necessarily the numbers on the scale we need to worry about; it's how fat is stored inside our bodies. What makes us unhealthy is excess fat in all the wrong places — protruding from the stomach and clustering around and even in our vital organs.

When fat accumulates in the arteries, our hearts are at especially grave risk. Yet we can't see the fat forming, so we don't necessarily make the connection. But as we'll see in the next section, a growing body of research suggests that some of our most prevalent and dangerous diseases seem to be tied to poor eating choices that affect that most vital of all our vital organs, the heart.

CHAPTER 11

Sugar And The Heart

FOR DECADES, WE HAVE TRIED to use what we know — or think we know — about cardiovascular disease to explain the many conditions that often precede it: obesity, diabetes, hypertension (high blood pressure), dyslipidemia (high LDL and low HDL cholesterol), elevated triglycerides, and atherosclerosis (stiffening of the arteries). When the heart has to work harder to pump blood throughout the body because of stiff arterial walls or buildups of fat and cholesterol in the arteries themselves, we run a much greater risk of suffering heart attacks, strokes, or other potentially fatal afflictions.

High blood pressure and clogged arteries jump out immediately as direct factors of heart problems, but what causes these initial conditions to develop is less certain. The lipid hypothesis — the dominant theory in cardiovascular research for the past fifty or so years — has pinned blame on dietary cholesterol and saturated fat. This may explain fatty buildups in the arteries but fails to account for all the symptoms of metabolic syndrome that so frequently lead up to cardiovascular events — particularly insulin resistance and diabetes. Type 2 diabetics are twice as likely to experience heart attacks or stroke as the rest of the population, but the lipid hypothesis primarily views insulin resistance as a symptom, rather than a potential cause, of heart disease itself. What if they both start from the same place?

The "sugar hypothesis" of heart disease starts with excess glucose-fructose consumption and explores how it eventually leads to cardiovascular problems. It recognizes that insulin resistance and de novo lipogenesis (the conversion of carbohydrates to fats in the liver from glucose and fructose, respectively) can build to dangerous heights that produce hypertension, dyslipidemia, and high blood pressure. And that those problems will eventually result in atherosclerosis and heart disease.

As we've seen, when refined sugars are metabolized in the body, glucose enters the bloodstream and fructose is sent to the liver for conversion. Once fructose is transformed from a dietary carbohydrate into a lipid, it needs to be transported via the bloodstream to its destined purpose: either used up as energy or stored in the body as fat for later energy use. Lipids, proteins, and cholesterols are all carried from the liver through the rest of the body in bundles called lipoproteins — but not all lipoproteins are created equally.

Good, Bad, And Worse

You've probably heard of good and bad cholesterol. They refer to two broad categories: high-density lipoproteins (HDL) and low-density lipoproteins (LDL). The more proteins per lipoprotein, the higher the density and the better for you. HDLs — "good" cholesterols — are swift, efficient lipoproteins that can clear through the arteries and even remove plaque and buildup along the way. LDLs ("bad" cholesterols) are heavy, sluggish, and prone to getting stuck in arterial walls. (This is a simplified breakdown, as both HDL and LDL cholesterol actually have good and bad factions to them; but for our purposes, we'll stick to the generalized "good" and "bad" definitions.) Enough LDLs backed up can cause the kind of blockage that leads to heart attacks, strokes, clotting, and aneurysms.

The lipoproteins are the *vehicles* for lipids. Different types of lipids prefer different types of lipoprotein-carrying systems. It used to be thought that saturated fats, like those found in fatty meat, promoted the formation of "bad" LDLs. But recent research shows that saturated fats increase HDLs more than LDLs (and mostly the good faction of LDL). Monounsaturated fats, found in vegetable oils and foods such as olives and avocados, also promote the formation of "good" HDLs. Research shows that it's trans fats and processed foods that are thought to produce the formation of "bad" LDLs.

Here's an important point about cholesterol: it's only produced by animals inside their bodies. There's no dietary cholesterol *in* any fruits or vegetables, but our bodies can produce cholesterol *from* them. So dietary cholesterol is only found in foods from other animals: meat, dairy, poultry, eggs, etc. And just as dietary fat does not necessarily cause bodily fat, dietary cholesterol does not necessarily translate into the cholesterol readings your doctor gives you. Between 85 and 90% of the cholesterol in our body is produced by the liver. Only a small fraction is influenced by diet.

Cholesterol is cholesterol; it's the way it's carried through the blood that makes the difference.

Fructose, the sweet part of refined sugars that acts like a lipid, prefers to be carried in the bloodstream via *very low-density lipoproteins* (VLDLs). Like the name suggests, these lipoprotein molecules are even bigger, bulkier, and more cumbersome than the "bad cholesterol" LDLs from trans fats. And it only gets worse: These fructose molecules are so demanding and particular about their lipoprotein vehicles that instead of breaking down into smaller pieces when there aren't enough VLDLs available, the fructose-lipids will clump together to form clusters known as triglycerides. But instead of using the carpool lane, these clusters are prone to causing traffic jams in the bloodstream and arteries.

High counts of triglycerides and high levels of LDLs in the blood make for an unusually high balance of lipids circulating through the body, a condition called dyslipidemia that is directly correlated with a greater chance of heart disease.

Fructose in particular seems to aggravate triglyceride production: men on an experimental high-fructose diet saw their triglyceride levels increase by 32% in just six weeks.[93] Additionally, excess amounts of insulin — like the kind seen in insulin resistance and type 2 diabetes — encourages the further production of triglycerides by the liver than under normal circumstances.

People who consume 15% or more of their daily calories from sugar (the equivalent of 24 ounces of soda in a 2,000-calorie diet) are up to *three times* more likely to exhibit high triglyceride levels, high LDLs, and low "good" HDLs than those who consume 5% or less of their calories from sugar every day.[94]

When large lipoprotein molecules and triglycerides accumulate in the bloodstream, it becomes more difficult for the heart to pump blood through the arteries. The harder the heart has to pump, the more strain it has to endure, which can eventually exhaust the muscles, especially if the strain is continuous for years on end. No one likes to be continuously overworked.

So this suggests that sugar is the real culprit, since half of people hospitalized with heart attacks have no cholesterol problems, and half of people with high cholesterol have no heart disease. And consider that for 95% of the population, dietary cholesterol has virtually no effect on cholesterol in the blood. In fact, cholesterol is important for cell functioning. Made in the liver, it makes up a major part of the membranes surrounding all cells. Communication between neurons in the brain depends on cholesterol. So, cholesterol might not be quite the bad guy it's been made out to be after all.

Under Pressure

Blood pressure readings are simply a measure of the amount of force exerted to move blood through the arteries; the higher the numbers, the harder the heart is working with every pump. One-third of Americans experience chronic high blood pressure, or hypertension, which is the single biggest reason for visits to doctors in the United States.

Many factors can influence the amount of blood pressure in our veins: genetics, stress, activity levels, and, of course, diet. The principal dietary suspect here is usually sodium, or, as it's typically found in our foods, salt. Salt's ability to retain moisture makes it an ideal preservative in prepackaged foods, but it also retains water inside our bodies, which increases the strain on the kidneys, arteries, and heart muscles. Sugar also has similar, though less pronounced, water-retention properties — so sugar and salt combined seem especially likely to raise blood pressure.

In laboratory studies, animals fed higher levels of sodium predictably experienced higher blood pressure readings; but when refined sugars were added to their diets, blood pressure levels rose even higher, no matter their sodium intake levels.[95] Diets (for humans) that are heavy in refined sugars that contain both glucose and fructose have been shown to produce significantly higher blood pressure levels than starch-based (i.e., pure glucose) diets.[96]

Sugar and sodium are particularly abundant in pre-packaged foods because they also happen to enhance the flavors of other ingredients; they bring out the tomato flavor of pasta sauce, for example, or the meat flavor of frozen meatballs. As with sugar, the high levels of sodium in our diets are cooked right in: more than 75% of all sodium consumed in America comes from the salt contained in processed or restaurant-prepared foods.

Caffeine is often another suspect in the aggravation of hypertension. However, the case seems circumstantial: there's little proven correlation between chronic hypertension and coffee or tea consumption, but there is a pronounced relationship between soft drink consumption and high blood pressure readings.[97] Sodas, soft drinks, and especially energy drinks pack a triple threat to the heart, with hefty levels of sugar, sodium, or caffeine — or often all three. A typical energy drink like Monster or Red Bull contains as much as 50 grams of sugar (or 200 calories' worth — twice the daily limit recommended by the American Heart Association), over 350mg of sodium (16% of the daily recommended value), and 160mg of caffeine, the equivalent of two strong cups of coffee. And that's only in one sixteen-ounce can that many people down on their morning commute.

Hypertension affects some 76.4 million Americans today, including a remarkable 3% of children and teens. Treatment for the condition averages $1,000 per afflicted person per year. Other related metabolic conditions are no better: though our methods of managing and controlling cholesterol and triglyceride levels have greatly improved in the past decade, the incidence of dyslipidemia has remained at a constant 34% of the population. Currently, one in four Americans over the age of 40 takes prescribed medication to manage lipid and cholesterol levels, usually in the form of statins. Statins are the number-one prescribed drug in America, even though their real efficacy and safety remains questionable within some medical circles. And these drugs can cost patients anywhere from $12 to $500 per month.

I don't deny that pharmaceuticals can save lives, but their focus is inevitably on the treatment of disease, not its prevention. After all, if no one needed drugs anymore to stay healthy, pharmaceutical companies would be out of business. But from a quality-of-life standpoint, preventing disease is always preferable to treating it, and out-of-balance cholesterol — like obesity, diabetes, and hypertension — is extremely preventable with the right tools and knowledge.

Meanwhile, rates of heart disease in the United States are projected to rise another 10% by 2030, and by then it's going to cost us triple the amount of money to manage every case.[98] The current methods of combating heart disease and metabolic syndrome — popping pills and curbing intakes of saturated fat, dietary cholesterol, or sodium — simply aren't working.

Relying on medicine to treat the symptoms after they arise isn't working, either. We're much better off stopping the symptoms of cardiovascular disease before they have a chance to start.

CHAPTER 12

AGEs, Aging, and Cancer

IT MIGHT BE IMPOSSIBLE TO stop the aging process, but what if you knew that eating too much sugar could make you age faster? Just as many parts of our bodies become stiff with age, so do our arteries. Our arterial walls will naturally lose some of their pliability and elasticity as we get older, no matter what we do. To an extent, atherosclerosis — the hardening of the artery walls — is a natural part of aging, the same as wrinkles or gray hairs. But just how quickly we get there is another matter.

Our bodies are full of cells that eagerly collect whatever we give them. The longer we're alive, the more junk we tend to accumulate inside of those cells, just like the far corners of a closet that never get cleaned out. It's called "junk food" for a reason: some of the less desirable aspects of our foods that enter the body may have no purpose and therefore no way to get used up, unlike the vitamins and nutrients we depend on to function. The "junk" of junk food just kind of sits there inside our cells, with nothing to do and nowhere to go. And the more of it we eat, the more it accumulates. It might be a tiny, infinitesimally gradual increase, but over time, such junk might collect so high within our cells that it actually overflows; the junk can spill over the cell walls and into the synapse gaps between neurons, blocking the important electrical signals that transmit information between nerve cells. The cells, full of junk, tend to lose some of their elasticity. When this kind of deterioration occurs in the arteries, it's part of what produces atherosclerosis. If it happens in skin cells, it produces wrinkles. If it happens in and between brain cells, it can cause dementia.

It's not just the junk food we eat: the buildup in cells throughout our lives comes from both internal and external sources, and some of it is as inevitable as breathing. But certain sources tend to aggravate buildup in the cells more than others; two particularly notorious insurgents are what's called free radicals and advanced glycation end-products (or the apt acronym, AGEs, for short).

Free radicals and AGEs both start as imbalanced molecules inside the body seeking to stabilize themselves, as all molecules do. Most molecules have an even number of electrons, but free radicals don't. This makes them highly charged and highly reactive with other molecules around them, as they attempt to swipe electrons from atoms around them in order to stabilize themselves.

AGEs are less about balance and more about convenience. AGEs are a synthesis of carbohydrate molecules and protein or lipid molecules; the smaller carbohydrates like hitching up to larger protein or fat molecules — which are abundant in our cell walls — and using them to get around, kind of like fleas on a dog. They also can distort the shape of the cells to the point where the cells can't function properly.

In this way, both AGEs and free radicals are major antagonists in the war of aging constantly going on throughout our bodies, and are especially key players in the battle known as oxidative stress. Oxidation is a chemical reaction between certain substances and, of course, oxygen, which is abundant in the air we breathe. Oxidation, or oxidative stress, is what causes iron to rust or bananas to turn brown. It's also happening inside of our cells, although we can't see it happening. Like the way rust builds on a car over the years, the change is almost imperceptible — but it's happening constantly, little by little.

Free radicals are an unavoidable part of life. They bring oxygen — and thus oxidation — into the body through such simple (and important) activities as regular breathing and exercise. Antioxidants (which you may have seen advertised on your fruit yogurt or juice, since they're especially abundant in foods like berries with vitamins C and E) are just that — molecules that fight oxidation. Or, if not fight, at least appease the free radicals by offering up a plentitude of spare electrons.

The formation of AGEs, on the other hand, requires the presence of simple sugars, most of which come from the foods we eat. Simple sugars are the basic carbohydrates that make up larger sugars, like glucose, fructose, and galactose (the milk sugar). AGEs form inside of us all the time as ingested carbohydrates find a protein or lipid to cling to for a free ride. But they can also form even before they enter the body whenever we cook foods with both fat and sugars. The caramelization of an onion as it's sautéed in butter, for example, is an active process of AGE formation and oxidation. We can see the change occur before our very eyes because the heat we use to cook with speeds up the process. The very same thing is what happens inside our bodies, only at a much lower heat, which makes it take a longer time. That lovely brown color of barbecued meat, baked apple crisp, even the crust of a loaf of bread — that's the same thing that happens to us. It's all due to AGEs.

Clearly it wouldn't be practical or enjoyable to try to avoid AGEs altogether. And thankfully, the body has natural ways of coping with these unwanted substances. A lot of AGEs simply get flushed out of the system with no harm done. Our body's capacity to do this is limited, though, and the more AGEs we consume or produce, the tougher it is to make sure they all get sent out. Some invariably get left behind, begetting the buildup of cell junk that essentially amounts to the aging process.

It's logical to infer that our rate of aging can be determined in part by the rate at which free radicals and AGEs accumulate in our cells, which in turn can be impacted by our diets. Because AGEs are made up of bound-together simple sugars and proteins, the more sugars we ingest, the more likely AGEs are to form. The consumption of refined sugars, like table sugar or high-fructose corn syrup, provides exactly the kind of fodder for AGE formation that fuels oxidative stress. Fructose in particular is *really* good at finding protein molecules to cling to: these simple sugars are known to produce AGEs at *ten times* the rate of glucose. High amounts of fructose and glucose combined can also foster the production of free radicals within the body, even within hours of ingesting soft drinks or other sugar-dense foods.[99]

Life-Shortening — Literally

One recent study brought results that are as groundbreaking as they are straightforward.

The research looked at telomeres, the sequences of DNA at the end of our chromosomes. Telomeres shorten with each cell division. Eventually the telomere length runs out and the cell can no longer rejuvenate, leading to cellular death. It is estimated that humans can live approximately 122 years if telomere length is optimally maintained.

Inflammation, stress, and sugar have been shown to accelerate the rate at which telomeres shorten — essentially speeding up the aging process. Premature telomere-shortening is associated with heart disease, obesity, diabetes, cancer, and dementia.

A study in the *American Journal of Public Health* (reported on Oct. 16, 2014 and authored by Sara N. Bleich, Colleen L. Barry, Tiffany L. Gary-Webb, and Bradley J. Herring) was the first study to show that sugar-sweetened beverages are associated with telomere-shortening and cellular aging. Elizabeth Blackburn, who received the Nobel Prize in 2009 for her work relating to the topic, calculated that the daily consumption of 20 ounces of a sugar-sweetened beverage was associated with 4.6 years of accelerated biological aging. That's comparable to the negative effects of smoking.

Good nutrition, though, could play an opposite role. Studies are now evaluating nutritional intake as a means to slow down telomere shortening, repair damaged telomeres, and actually lengthen telomeres.

But for now, it's a remarkable finding. A 20-ounce soda a day may shave off an average of almost half a decade from a person's life.

Diet and Dementia

People with diabetes, as we've talked about before, tend to have chronically high levels of glucose in the bloodstream at any given time. This makes them especially prone to the development of free radicals and AGEs because those molecules are constantly abundant, always looking for a way to get by. In turn, diabetics are more likely to develop diseases explicitly related to aging and oxidation, such as atherosclerosis and dementia.

In fact, people living with type 2 diabetes have twice the risk of developing Alzheimer's disease, the most prevalent form of dementia, than do non-diabetics. Alzheimer's currently affects one in eight Americans over the age of 65, and one in two over age 85. Because it's about the accumulation of junk (potentially, anyway — no one truly understands the precise causes or mechanics yet), the chance of developing Alzheimer's increases with age. But the preliminary risk factors at any age highly resemble those associated with heart disease, including hypertension, high cholesterol, and insulin resistance.

The same dysfunctional mechanisms that will strain and weaken the heart seem to potentially affect the brain as well. Blood flow is important for the brain's functioning, and if the heart can't do its job well, neither can the brain. Neural pathways of the brain can be damaged over time by free radicals and AGEs, and that damage to the neural system might lead to the types of memory loss and cognitive decline associated with Alzheimer's and other forms of dementia.

The accumulation of AGEs is a natural part of aging; dementia is not. Dementia might be viewed as an extreme case of AGE buildup, where blockages in the brain cause functional disruptions similar to the way blockages in the arteries contribute to heart disease. Blockages in the brain — known as senile plaques — often found in Alzheimer's patients tend to contain a high concentration of AGEs, which clump together between cell synapses and obstruct the normal flow of information.[100]

Another type of dementia, vascular dementia, is caused by multiple series of tiny strokes (the stoppage of blood flow) in the vessels of the brain. Vascular dementia is a frequent complication of type 2 diabetes and can occur in Alzheimer's disease as well. The brain's blood vessels are made vulnerable to these kinds of strokes because of oxidative stress; free radicals and AGEs alike make for a slow process of deterioration that wears on cognitive health and functionality.

As the American population ages, especially the Baby Boomer generation that has long been raised on sugar, the increasing rates of dementia may prove more than our current medical system is prepared to handle. By 2050, an estimated 20% of all people 65 or older will likely experience some form of clinical dementia, and the projected cost of associated care exceeds $1.2 trillion dollars.[101] Seventy percent of the medical support for senior citizens with dementia would be provided through tax-funded programs like Medicaid and Medicare, which even today experience a significant financial burden; some estimates suggest the money behind such programs could run out within the next ten years.

One in three Americans over age 65 will die with some form of dementia. If the theory of oxidative stress as the source behind many cases of Alzheimer's and other diseases of aging is correct, we could likely prevent or at least delay some instances of dementia through diet alone. An AGE-conscious diet — low in simple sugars (*especially* fructose) and with reasonable limits on the amount of cooking-formed AGEs found in caramelized or browned foods — may be able to decrease AGE levels circulating in the blood by as much as 30-40%.[102] And minimizing the effects of free radicals through a diet rich in antioxidants like vitamin E may prove beneficial in preventing Alzheimer's and other forms of dementia.[103]

More Diet-Related Disease

The foods we eat don't just nourish us from the mouth down; for better or worse, everything we ingest becomes brain food in one way or another.

The high density of cells inside the brain help us think, feel, and reason — but it also makes our body's most complex organ especially vulnerable to the type of damage inflicted by AGEs and free radicals. Wherever there are cells — and there are about 100 trillion of them throughout every inch of our bodies — there exists the potential for molecular damage. AGEs have even been potentially implicated in the formation of certain types of cancer in the colon and liver, where the inflammation caused by oxidative stress may become extreme enough to produce an abnormal growth of cells resulting in tumors.[104, 105] The electron-swapping games of free radicals can cause organ tissue or DNA molecules within cells to mutate haphazardly into cancerous cells that then multiply throughout the body. Known carcinogens, such as tobacco smoke and UV rays, are also potent aggravators of AGE and free radical formation; it may be the same mechanisms of oxidative stress that drive cancer, regardless of its source.

An increasing amount of studies are positing correlations between AGEs, sugars, and cancer. Even though we tend to think of cancer as striking randomly and unexpectedly — a bad luck of the draw — the World Cancer Research Fund estimates that one-third of all cancer cases can be attributed to diet and nutrition habits, which means they could have possibly been prevented. Some medical communities think that as many as half of all cancers are preventable.[106]

Cancer development may be caused by AGEs or free radicals, or it may have to do directly with sugar itself: consumption of refined sugars correlates positively with the risk of developing esophageal cancer, leukemia, pleural tumors, and bladder and intestinal cancers in all people, and with breast cancer in post-menopausal women.[107, 108] Insulin resistance is further associated with colon cancer and endometrial (uterine) cancer.[109, 1110]

The cancers most highly linked with diet are diseases of either the gastrointestinal tract (esophagus, intestines, colon) or of parts of the body that are closely regulated by hormones (white blood cells, reproductive organs). Hormonal imbalances, such as the chronic overproduction of insulin, may be associated with these malicious growths, stimulating and even accelerating the growth of malignant tumor cells.[111]

Some cancerous cells have insulin receptors on their surface. As insulin bonds with the receptors, it tells the tumor to start consuming glucose to grow. While there's some debate about the relationship between sugar and cancer, a growing number of researchers believe that sugar can promote the growth of cancer cells.

Cancer is the second-leading cause of death in the United States, right behind heart disease. Over 1,665,000 new cases are diagnosed every year in the United States; more than 1,600 people die from cancer every day.[112] I don't mean to say that cancer is the person's own fault, or that if we kick sugar all cancer will be over forever — we're far from understanding the direct relations of cause and effect in cancer, and the many types of cancer vary so tremendously that we may never be able to cure them all with one fell swoop. But there are certain types of cancer irrefutably linked with the foods we eat, and taking a hard look at our diet could prevent a lot of tragic, unnecessary deaths. Imagine if we could eradicate those 1 in 3 cases of diet-related cancers: we'd save almost 200,000 lives every year, not to mention a large part of $30 billion in annual health care expenditures.

When Enough Is Enough

Every pack of cigarettes in the United States today comes with a label warning of the risk of cancer, death, or heart disease from the use of tobacco. Yet the number of deaths in the U.S. attributable to our diets and the way we eat is now on par with deaths caused from smoking. Of the top seven leading causes of death in the U.S., sugar is complicit in at least five: heart disease, diabetes, stroke, cancer, and Alzheimer's disease.

I've tried here to summarize the amount of medical evidence building against sugar. Researchers and practitioners in the medical field tend to stick to their own specialty, making it difficult sometimes to draw a big picture from all the smaller pieces. But the picture we have here is clear, impressive, and immensely troubling. Is it right to consider sugar safe? Should we even be calling it a food? When you consider the science, experts from many fields seem to draw the same conclusion: that sugar is a slow-acting poison. From where I stand, it's much more a toxin than dessert topping.

With enough time and enough dosage, sugar is inherently damaging to our blood, hearts, brains, and organs. Every smoker knows that tobacco kills.

But does every soda drinker know they're voluntarily taking on the same sort of risk? We deserve to know what the potential consequences of our actions might be, especially when we're socialized to think that sugar is nothing but sweet.

The question now is: Can we stop — even if we want to?

CHAPTER 13

The Birth of Cavities

FIVE HUNDRED YEARS AGO, physicians were already warning us that sugar "makes the teeth blunt and makes them decay."[113] Despite the clear correlation, most people continue to eat sugar as much as they like. When we pick up a chocolate or a soda, some of us may fleetingly consider the implications on our weight or health. But rarely do we think about the relationship between food and our teeth.

It seems almost old-fashioned now to say "Sugar will rot your teeth out!" but — left unchecked — it's true. Today, modern dentistry, oral health care, and the fluoridation of public water systems have greatly diminished the prevalence of tooth decay and cavities, but that doesn't erase the fact that sugar is extremely likely to promote them. And even though they are now largely preventable, dental cavities remain the most common form of chronic disease among children.[114] So accustomed to and dependent on sugar are we that, rather than give it up, we've actually invented new technologies and systems to treat the consequences — but not the causes.

Before refined sugar became widespread, before the sugarcane colonization of the Americas, dental cavities in European cultures were extremely rare. Even up to the time of Queen Elizabeth I, cavities were almost exclusively seen among only the very rich — probably from "their too great use of sugar," as one traveling German wrote of England in 1598.[115] Elizabeth herself was known to have rotted, black teeth and a great penchant for sweets. As sugar became more common and prevalent, in Europe and America alike, so too did the rate of dental problems: by the 1960s, the average American teenager already had between four and nine decayed, missing, or filled teeth. Studies at the same time in England found no difference in the rate of cavities between 13-year-old boys who did or did not brush their teeth, but those who ate more sweets in either group had significantly more dental problems.[116] Throughout the world, even today, the availability and prevalence of sugars can accurately predict a correlative rate of dental cavities by country.[117]

Cavities develop when growths of bacteria erode the surface of the teeth. Normally, our saliva is sufficient to clear off food bacteria. But certain types of foods, like sugars and simple carbohydrates, encourage the growth of bacteria more so than other foods. Inadequate nutrition can even affect the properties of saliva, rendering it less powerful or efficient at cleaning the teeth.[118] And when foods get stuck in our teeth, as things like sticky candies and soft white bread are wont to do, it increases the exposure time between the sugars and the tooth enamel, increasing the potential for erosion and decay.

There's an urban legend that allowing a human tooth to sit in a glass of cola for twenty-four hours will cause it to dissolve. True or not, most people aren't holding soda in their mouths for that long. But a repetitive stream of contact, like sipping on a drink all day and eating sweets, in effect exposes the teeth to an equally cumulative amount of potential sugar decay, especially over years of habitual drinking.[119] Soft drink consumption is positively correlated with dental cavities or decay in both children and adults, and a long history of studies shows a direct relationship between sugar intake and cavity rates. [120, 121, 122]

In all the years of human existence, never before have we ever had such frequent and common dental problems — nor, ironically, such advanced technology in and knowledge of oral hygiene. Studies of Anglo-Saxon remains spanning over 2,000 years — from the Iron Age of BCE to Medieval times — show no significant differences in the rate of cultural tooth decay, even though oral hygiene practices were poor or nonexistent throughout all of these years.[123] Cavities only began to increase after the 1700s, reaching critical proportions by the twentieth century in Western countries; frequently, the only treatment was to pull out the rotted teeth. In the United States, many men were turned down for military service in both World Wars because they failed to meet the required minimum possession of six opposing teeth.[124]

Mottled Teeth

One of the first major breakthroughs in public preventive dentistry came, ironically, from a bunch of people with brown teeth. In the early 1900s, oral practitioners were baffled by a strange case where the entire population of Colorado Springs started developing mottled stains on their teeth. They weren't rotting, though — in fact, they were remarkably strong and resistant teeth, not a cavity among them. Eventually they traced the cause back to the town's water supply, which was unusually high in mineral fluoride. This got scientists thinking and researching, as scientists do, and a few decades later public fluoridation was born.

Too much fluoride might stain your teeth, like the people of Colorado Springs, but low enough amounts can prevent cavity development without any major staining. The Colorado case offered a ready-made example of how to get it out to the people, too: just put it in their drinking water.

Before then, few people knew what fluoride was or that it could have any application to dental health. Today, two-thirds of American tap water is supplemented with fluoride, and more than 90% of commercial toothpastes are fluoridated as well. The Centers for Disease Control and Prevention called public water fluoridation "one of the ten great public health achievements of the 20th century;"[125] it has effectively reduced the incidence of cavities and tooth decay in the general population, and especially youth, by as much as 50%.

Even so, 1 in 4 U.S. children between the ages of 2 and 5 — and 1 in 2 children aged 12 to 15 — are still affected by dental caries. Fluoride may be considered a preventive treatment, but it continues to ignore the principal root cause behind the still prevalent trend of modern dental problems: sugar. Personal and professional administration of oral health and hygiene is so advanced and useful that, of people who brush their teeth once a day, there is no relationship between any type of food intake and the subsequent risk of dental cavities — *except sugar*.[126] Despite care, despite education, despite fluoridation, cavities remain far more rampant than they were even 200 years ago, or ever before in the entirety of human history, all because of our modern sweet tooth.

We may pat ourselves on the back for the great public health solution that is fluoridation. And it's certainly nothing to scoff at: every public dollar spent on public fluoridation saves an average $38 in personal dental care bills.[127] But imagine the savings potential if we could just curb sugar consumption. Sugar is what makes us susceptible to cavities and decay in the first place; without sugar, we wouldn't need fluoride.

Giving up sweets isn't nearly as fun, easy, or feasible an option — not when we can count on medicine and technology, like dentists and municipal water systems, to get around the problems for us. Dental damage is one of the oldest, best-proved, and most commonly known ill effects of sugar consumption, yet we rarely ever think about it anymore because we simply trust that modern medicine will be able to fix it for us.

Fluoride was supposed to be the silver bullet of oral health, but even that couldn't fix America's rotting sweet teeth. It only put a Band-Aid of damage control over what's clearly a much larger epidemic.

Not So Easy

As successful as the fluoride story is, it sets a dangerous precedent when it comes to sugar. The lesson is that we can eat whatever we want and as much as we like because, eventually, science and technology will figure out how to make better any harm we might have done to ourselves along the way. It's not true. There's no magic pill or substance we can slip into the drinking well to save us from obesity or heart disease. There's no quick fix to dementia or cancer.

We as a society can't just wait around until medical technology comes up with the answers for us. We can't assume that there ever will be answers to give. We have to look closer to home. We have to take responsibility for the problems we've brought upon ourselves.

But that's just it — we are the problem. It's easy enough to say we'll cut back on sugar, but actually doing it, physically and mentally, is another question.

A peek inside our brains — our brains on sugar — shows the epic tug-of-war waging in our minds that can make it feel as if we *need* sugar, even when we don't.

PART IV:

Sugarholics

Your Brain on Sugar

CHAPTER 14

The Evolutionary Pull

SWEETNESS IS A TASTE ALMOST UNIVERSALLY ADORED. Around the globe and throughout time, it seems that humans are biologically hardwired to love the sight, smell, and taste of sugars.

There are a couple of good evolutionary reasons for this. Sweetness signifies the availability of safe and nutritious calories: in nature, no plant is both sweet-tasting and acutely poisonous. Back when humans roamed the earth as nomadic hunter-gatherers, a sugary plant meant a safe plant. Sweetness comes in the form of carbohydrates, which equates to food energy that's readily available to nourish our cells and quell hunger. Stocking up on carbohydrates served as a safeguard against starvation and was a key to our survival as a species. Sugarcane in its whole form, the most calorie-dense plant on earth, was the ultimate find for our hungry ancestors.

These days, we all know how many sweets a typical child can pack away. Most soft drinks are formulated to suit the taste of adults, but children, when given a choice, will more often prefer sugary drinks that are *twice* as sweet as a typical soda.[128] Again, it goes back to the body's demands for calories: growing children require more energy, and those experiencing growth spurts may crave even more sweets. The intensity of a child's sweet tooth tends to taper off toward the end of adolescence, as soon as most of the body's growing is complete. But as most of us can attest to, a strongly developed taste for sweets tends to carry through to adulthood.

It's not just the calories that make sweets so irresistible. Every time we eat, it triggers a vast, complicated response system in the part of our brains that rewards us for our behavior. This happens for all foods, but some — like sugar — are especially adept at stimulating the feel-good response network that comes with eating. It's human instinct on the most basic level, wired into us: when we eat, we feel good, so we're more likely to do it again — and thus more likely to survive.

In fruits and other naturally sweet foods, sugars are accompanied by a host of life-supporting vitamins and minerals. But our candy bars and soft drinks? Not so much. But since we've managed to extract pure sugars from whole plants, our evolutionary failsafe has backfired. Once upon a time, foods such as a bush of wild blueberries were available only for a short season or in small quantities. Now, even sweeter "finds" are all over the place — in every grocery aisle and every vending machine across the country — and our brains still trigger us to go after them. The problem is knowing when — and how — to stop.

Learning To Like It

At the same time, our personal preference for how much sweetness we can tolerate or enjoy is actually an acquired taste. We all acclimate to a culture of available sweetness. If you've ever abstained from sugar for a stretch of time or managed to keep on a low-carb or dessert-free diet, you may have experienced this phenomenon first-hand: when (inevitably, it seems) we break our diets and dive into a piece of cake again, it can be startling just how sweet that frosting tastes, when only last month it wouldn't have seemed anything out of the ordinary.

When we eat sugar, we feel rewarded. But the more sugar we eat, the harder it is to generate the same type of reward response. We build a physical tolerance in our taste buds and, mentally, we crave increasingly more just to satisfy that sweet tooth. It's no surprise that the food culture around us is becoming increasingly sugar-steeped; even our fruits are being genetically engineered and bred to taste sweeter. Often, though, that increase in sugars comes at the expense of nutrients and fiber.

In modern American culture, we get doused in sugar from the moment we're born — quite literally. The mother's breast milk that nourishes us in our infancy contains naturally occurring milk sugars (mostly glucose plus galactose, or lactose) that make it sweet, but mass-produced infant formulas that try to mimic human milk often get their sweetness from refined sugars containing glucose and/or fructose. This spells potential trouble for our diet and metabolism early on: several studies have linked the practice of formula-feeding instead of breast-feeding as a predictor of childhood obesity and have linked formula use with the development of a higher tolerance threshold for sweetness later on in life.[129, 130]

As you may know if you've raised a child, babies often have to be exposed to new foods, especially savory ones like beans or vegetables, a dozen times or more before they'll readily accept them. But if the food is sweet, infants will typically take to it immediately. For just this reason, many ready-made store-bought brands of jarred, pureed baby foods contain high amounts of added sugars — sometimes accounting for as much as 75% of the meal's total calories.[131]

And it doesn't stop there: once kids graduate to solid foods, many of the highest-sugar products available on store shelves — cereals, fruit juices, snacks, and desserts — will be marketed directly toward them (or their parents, who are the ones doing the purchasing). Kids not only learn to like, want, and ask their parents for such foods, but they even come to think that's what kids are *supposed* to be eating. These consumption patterns and preferences established early on in life are likely to form habits and tastes that follow us through adulthood, sometimes devastatingly so: children who are overweight or obese by age five are apt to remain that way for the rest of their lives.[132]

By the time we're old enough to leave the parental nest and make food choices of our own, many of us will already be well accustomed to a sugar-saturated diet — so much so that we usually fail to notice just how ubiquitous sugars are in our shopping carts or the physical and psychological cravings that drive us to keep consuming sugars again and again. Yet even if we do try to take control over our sugar diets — for health or weight reasons, for example — we often find ourselves fatigued, irritable, or even depressed in such a way that, it seems, only a pint of ice cream or a big slice of chocolate cake could cure us.

Imagine yourself in the middle of your workday, confronted with a tray of your favorite sweets: brownies, doughnuts, candies — pick your poison. Even if you're well rested, comfortably fed, and reasonably cheerful, would you be able to resist taking a bite? And what if you're tired, hungry, or grumpy — does the urge strike you even more? Sugar doesn't only taste good, it feels good. Our drive for sweets isn't just about physical nourishment; it's also about emotional nourishment. It's called "comfort food" for a reason.

Like all foods, sugars have the ability to affect our mood and cognition by acting on the mental and emotional systems of the brain and nervous system — only, just like we saw with the body's metabolism, refined sugars tend to cause reactions in a quicker and bigger way. Our diets influence the internal processes that regulate our happiness, stress levels, perceptions of pain, and overall mood, and sugar habits can really wreak havoc with the steady balance of these systems. In turn, these mental states can have a tremendous impact — possibly even more so than physical hunger or nutrition needs — over our food cravings.

We don't merely eat to live. We also live to eat. We eat in times of celebration or in times of sadness, in pain and in love, in sickness and in health. Food is not just about energy — it's also about living life. Food is a major part of our cultural identities, of rituals and traditions that can carry a heavy emotional meaning in our day-to-day experiences. And that food culture is changing in ways that we can't always control.

We all *know* that vegetables are healthier for us than cupcakes. But we still eat the cupcake, even if — *especially* if — we're trying very hard not to. It's difficult enough to try to go an entire day without eating sugars, much less thinking about them and craving them when we don't have them. Restrain yourself from that tray of your favorite goodies long enough, and it might start to drive you mad. The cravings might be so intense that you'll wonder: *Am I addicted to sugar?* If the brain could answer back, it would give you a resounding *Yes.*

CHAPTER 15

Sugar Smack

THE BRAIN LIKES TO REWARD US for good behavior. Even the simplest of tasks, like eating, keeping warm, reproducing, and socializing with other human beings, will trigger a wave of feel-good hormones — the brain's way of saying, "Good job! You've kept yourself and the human species alive for another day — we should try that again sometime!" When we're rewarded in this way, we're more likely to do these tasks again — not unlike the way a dog will perform tricks in return for treats.

Most of these rewards come in the form of a hormone called dopamine, which is crucial to our survival. Dopamine is what gives us motivation to live, eat, and simply get out of bed morning after morning. Scientists have done studies on dopamine in animals where their receptors for the hormone had been cut off; the poor creatures starved to death simply because they had no will to eat or seek out food.[133] Food consumption is a major trigger of dopamine in the brain, but different kinds of foods have different effects. Some, like leafy greens, don't stimulate too much dopamine, while really delicious foods or foods that we try (and like) for the first time will pour out a lot.

The naturally occurring sugars found inside of fruits and certain grains appear to be major triggers for dopamine, although — just like with our digestive system — fibers and waters keep the release slow, steady, and balanced at appropriate levels. When we isolate and refine those sugars, as in table sugar, high-fructose corn syrup, fruit sugars, syrups, and the rest, we essentially maximize the dopamine-stimulating potential. Those high and sudden spikes of dopamine from refined sugars generate brief surges of well-being, confidence, and alertness — what you might call a "sugar high."

If this starts to make sugar sound like a drug, that's because this is exactly how most drugs work on the brain, too. The feel-good mechanisms of drugs like cocaine, alcohol, heroin, and methamphetamines all operate through the same system, the dopamine reward system, launching cascades of hormones that feel good for a while and then, when their effects wear off, leave users craving more.

After a lot of repeated use, the dopamine surges — from drugs or sugars alike — stop feeling like a "high" and start feeling just normal. The body becomes acclimated to high levels of dopamine hanging around, and so the thrill wanes — unless the doses of dopamine (and the accompanying stimulant) are increased even more. Greater and greater amounts are required just to feel the same kick or high. This is precisely how a *tolerance* to a substance of any kind develops, and the cycle can continue to escalate until it spins out of control. Building tolerance is a dangerous stepping stone to addiction; it can mess with the brain's normal operations to the point where addicts are no longer able to function without their drug of choice providing the necessary flow of dopamine for basic daily task rewards.

This is another instance where the body's amazing capacity to adapt to its surroundings backfires, at least when it comes to drugs and addiction. Much like the way cells in the body can stop reacting to insulin and cause obesity and diabetes, cells in the brain may eventually stop reacting to repetitive high doses of dopamine. The chronic over-stimulation of dopamine receptors from drug abuse will lead the brain to make attempts at normalization; it does this by closing off the places on the cells where dopamine typically lands. Thus, these raging hormones are given fewer opportunities to make contact and have an effect. But when these receptor sites close, they're closed all the time — so it takes greater amounts of dopamine to have even a small effect. What once felt so great now might just feel okay or normal, and it'll take higher and higher doses to feel rewarded again. In addiction terms, we call this stage of use *dependence.*

Pleasure Pathway and Addiction

The ventral tegmental area (VTA) of the brain releases dopamine that binds to dopamine receptors. This is the reward center of the brain involved in pleasure and consumption. It is the same area of the brain that lights up with exposure to alcohol, amphetamines, cocaine, marijuana, sex, and gambling. When we consume sugar, it is this area that is responsible for the resulting "sugar high." Tolerance results when, after repeated stimulation, the dopamine receptors need more dopamine to experience the same level of reward or pleasure. This is the first step in addiction.[134]

When we are full from a meal, leptin (the "I'm full" hormone) slows down and blocks the release of dopamine, which curtails further consumption. In the accompanying diagram, this is denoted by the negative symbol, which corresponds to the negative feedback signal sent out by the ventral tegmental area. Normal levels of insulin also aid in this process by clearing dopamine from the synaptic areas.

However, with excessive production of insulin (hyperinsulinemia from overconsumption of sugar), leptin is blocked, resulting in a cessation of the negative feedback loop (denoted by the positive sign). More and more dopamine is released to the reward center and less of the dopamine is removed from the area. Now, the reward center is in overdrive and consumption continues unabated, resulting in overeating and obesity.

Remember, no one chooses to be addicted to sugar. No one chooses to be obese. Instead, we can blame an altered biochemical pathway that normally protects us and keeps us in balance.

The same caveats from the earlier diagram applies to this next series of graphs as well. Remember, the biological processes involved are very complex and this is simply an overview to aid in gaining a better understanding of the material. It, too, would flow the same if one has a *leptin resistance.*

Healthy Pleasure Pathway   ## Unhealthy Pleasure Pathway

Healthy Pleasure Pathway	Unhealthy Pleasure Pathway
Consume Food	Consume Food
⬇	⬇
Normal Insulin	Excessive Insulin
⬇	✖
Leptin	Leptin
⬇	⬇
VTA (Ventral Tegmental Area)	VTA (Ventral Tegmental Area)
⬇ ⊖	⬇ ⊕
Dopamine	Dopamine

Reward/Pleasure

Always Seeking
Reward/Pleasure
(i.e. Food Consumption)

⬤ = Dopamine Molecule

Another problem here is that tolerance and dependency put the user in a double bind. If, after a long while, the dopamine stimulators are drastically cut back (say, in an attempt to quit), the cells' receptor gates will still remain closed for a while. So even though the actual amount of dopamine circulating the system might be normal, it has no way of making an impact. The same amount of dopamine that keeps a non-user happy and carefree is useless to a recovering addict. The brain will feel deprived of dopamine, and will send out uncomfortable signals to the rest of the body to tell it so: anxiety, depression, headaches, nausea, and shakiness are all hallmark signs of *withdrawal.* Eventually, the body will re-acclimate to normal amounts of dopamine and re-open all of the usual receptor gates, but not without a lot of time and a good deal of suffering.

Tolerance, dependency, and withdrawal are three defining markers of any kind of substance addiction, especially ones that work on the brain's reward system. A spoonful of sugar might not have the same immediate, pronounced effects on dopamine production as, say, hard drugs like cocaine or heroin, but enough use over long periods of time can gradually cause the same kind of neurological mutations that lead to dependency and addiction.

To come out and call refined sugar a "drug" might seem far-fetched, but their essence is essentially the same: drugs and sugar are both concentrated forms of the stimulating properties of plants. Cocaine comes from the coca leaf; alcohol from distilled grains; heroin and morphine from the opium poppy; sugar from cane, beets, corn and other plants. The ability to take in large amounts of stimulants at once is what overwhelms the neurological system and is what gives drugs and sugars their appeal. Just like you couldn't get high on poppy seeds or drunk off of wheat, you don't get quite the same reaction from eating an apple as you do from refined sugars. It's the stimulants that our reward system craves, pure and simple.

It all begs the question: Should sugar be classified as a drug? Could a commonplace baking ingredient really be more of a narcotic?

The Case for Reclassifying

The potential for addiction is a compelling reason to qualify any substance as a drug that ought to be regulated or controlled. Food addiction in general is still a controversial idea, but it's one that's been gaining a lot of traction in medical and psychological fields over the past few decades. Before 1988, the term was virtually unheard of; but since 2009, hundreds of articles have appeared in scholarly and medical journals on the subject every year. The more research done, the more damning the evidence: foods, especially sugar, can have just as prominent effects on the inner workings of the brain as drugs, alcohol, and addictive behaviors like sex and gambling.

Most studies up to this point have been done on animals, especially lab rats, since it's not exactly ethical to subject humans to potentially harmful addictions. In many studies, animals given intermittent access to a sucrose (table sugar) drink solution will display all the signs of dopamine hyperactivity, including binging (which we'll talk about in humans later), tolerance, dependency, and subsequent withdrawal. In one 21-day experiment, the rats willingly tripled their sucrose intake from start to finish.[135] Other studies comparing the appeal of sugar and cocaine show that the animals will physically work just as hard for either reward[136] — and one even found that rats *prefer* Oreos to cocaine.[137]

We can't always apply findings from animal experiments to humans. But maybe there's a reason we joke about being "chocoholics" or call little sugary snacks "addictive." It's hard to say for sure because few of us are ever removed from sugar long enough to question whether our cravings are a harmless indulgence or a sign of dependency.

There are people who describe themselves as true food addicts and seek help for it. They often report a lost sense of control over their eating habits as well as withdrawal symptoms like depression, anxiety, and irritability, especially when cutting back on or abstaining from sugars.[138]

Because no hormone operates alone, other forces of the body might actually exacerbate the dopamine issue when it comes to sugars. Insulin and leptin, the tag-team force that regulate our digestive and blood glucose systems, are also involved in clearing out excess dopamine with meals — part of the cue to signify when we've had enough to eat. Consequently, a person who is insulin-resistant, and therefore also leptin-resistant, might also be over-stimulating dopamine receptors, since the cue for dopamine to clear out

—"Go home, the party's over" — doesn't get passed along properly. So not only do insulin-resistant people eat more before they start to feel full, they'll also keep receiving the feel-good dopamine rewards as they overeat.

Clearly, obesity is not just a biological issue; it's a *psychological* one, too. Eating is not just physical, but mental — something that most quick-and-dirty diet and exercise plans don't take into account. As common as obesity is in the United States (remember, two in three adults are overweight or obese), a stigma and prejudice associated with fatness in our culture still persists. People who are overweight are more likely to experience discrimination in the workplace, educational settings, and social settings, and may additionally face bias in medical and legal treatment.[139] On top of any potential haywire brain programming caused by sugars, overweight people are also stigmatized and ostracized by society, leading to high rates of depression, anxiety, and low self-esteem. Binge-eating is most likely to occur after a discriminatory experience[140] — and with dopamine at the ready, it's not hard to see why. If sugar's the problem in the first place, then it's also the crutch, the quick fix, the Band-Aid solution. It may make us feel good temporarily, but in the long run it causes more problems.

Sugar is a potent — and addictive — form of self-medication. It affects not only the reward system of the brain but also chemical signals that regulate mood (via the hormone serotonin), stress (with cortisol), and pain (via endorphins). Overall, sugar is quite the booster; but with too much use, it's bound to become an emotional crutch that's both necessary and devastating to our mental health.

CHAPTER 16

Less Pain, More Gain

HAVE YOU EVER WAVED HELLO to someone you thought you knew on the street, only to find out they're a complete stranger? The same kind of thing happens to the neurons in the brain if we use opiates, a class of drugs that includes morphine, heroin, and other narcotics. But obviously, the effects are a lot more sinister. Opiates look exactly like some of the brain's naturally produced communicators called endorphins, which are released to induce pleasure during certain vital activities (eating, sex) or with prolonged physical exertion to reduce pain and foster a kind of euphoria. (High-endurance athletes or marathoners who talk about a "runner's high" are getting a rush of endorphins attempting to disassociate the brain from the physical stress and pain going on in the body.)

To our brain cells, natural endorphins and drug opiates look so similar that they don't just wave hello, mistaking the latter for the former; they invite the opiates into their homes and allow them to use their best silver. Really, opiates are more like con men, going along with the trick in order to get what they want. Opiates can latch onto endorphin landing sites in the brain, triggering the same types of pleasure, painlessness, and euphoria the body usually reserves only for special occasions.

As with dopamine, endorphins are part of the behavioral reward system that congratulates us for simply managing to survive from day to day. Carbohydrate-rich foods like fruits and potatoes are especially good at triggering endorphin release, so imagine the rush that comes from a straight shot of pure, refined sugar.[141]

True, sugar stimulates natural endorphins, unlike the opiate drug mimickers. But the similarities are worth noting. Refined sugars and drugs are both concentrated stimulants that can produce much larger effects than any kind of naturally occurring food or intense activity could. Not only do you get the reward without working for it, but you can control when that reward comes by indulging in your endorphin-booster of choice as often as you want. In this sense, the endorphin high that comes from refined sugars should be seen as "artificial," too; the brain is tricked into giving out rewards for behaviors (like obtaining vital nutrients from healthy foods) that haven't actually occurred. Sugars will literally let you have your cake and eat it, too — but not without consequence.

Opiates and other endorphin-inducing substances shouldn't be entirely and immediately discounted, though. Morphine, for example, has played a crucial role in medicine for hundreds of years as an effective analgesic (painkiller). But its potency and high risk for addiction have rendered it more of a last-resort measure. Instead, many medical researchers have turned to *sugar* as a potential painkiller alternative, especially for use with small children and infants. Sugar-coating a pacifier has long been known to ease teething pains, and giving sugar solutions to young boys undergoing circumcision has been shown to reduce crying by as much as 60%.[142]

Animal experiments have delved further into the connections between sugar and the numbing of physical pain. Lab rats given a drink containing 11.5% sugars (just slightly more concentrated than most soft drinks) unwittingly took twice as long to react to a scalding hot pad under their paws than did their water-fed counterparts.[143] The implications here aren't just medical. If we consume high amounts of sugar, day in and day out, what sensations are we missing? What pain are we trying to numb?

Psychological Hurt

It's not just physical pain that sugar (and opiates and endorphins) can alleviate. The same researchers testing sugared-up animals' reactions to physical pain from hot pads beneath their paws also measured the response to psychological pain. Newborn mice were randomly separated from their mothers and given either a sugary drink or plain water. The water-fed babies cried 300 times or more, while the sugar-fed ones only cried an average 75 times during the same period.[144]

We can draw correlations between sugar consumption and pain relief in humans, too. People who are prone to depression, seasonal affective disorder, or premenstrual syndrome often exhibit a higher preference and craving for sweets during negative mood states, and they report feeling a temporary emotional ease after eating sugary foods.[145] So-called "emotional eating," or eating in response to stress, anxiety, anger, or depression, is commonly associated with binge-eating, and binge-eating sugary foods in particular.[146] Whether we're conscious of the process or not, sugar plays with our emotions.

As you might expect, the habitual use of artificial high-endorphin stimulants — opiate drugs and sugar alike — can permanently alter the brain's chemistry. That pattern of tolerance, dependency, and withdrawal can occur when endorphin sites are routinely over-stimulated, causing the brain to shut down receptor gates and the body to crave more endorphins just to maintain a sense of normalcy. After long periods of use, the brains of rats on a sugar diet and those of rats on a morphine diet end up looking remarkably similar.[147]

In part because of the endorphin system's close relationship with mechanisms of pain and pain relief, the withdrawal symptoms that often accompany opiate addiction recovery are notoriously brutal. Even comparatively minor abuse can cause cravings, anxiety, irritability, depression, and lethargy. The same patterns appear with sugar withdrawal as well. Lab rats addicted to morphine and lab rats addicted to sugar come out looking just the same. They develop severe tremors and hide in corners, teeth chattering. They'll barely muster the will or energy to swim to safety when placed in a pool of water. A full two weeks after the animals' sugar supply is cut off, they'll keep coming back to the button that used to give them their fix, often more times than ever before.[148]

Human sugar withdrawal isn't so easy to study or measure. As long as we keep consuming sugar on a regular basis, we may never notice the signs of withdrawal or recognize them for what they truly are. When we feel sluggish at work or when we're craving something sweet, it's incredibly easy to acquire a fix of sugar and make the symptoms disappear without a second thought. But if you've ever earnestly tried to stave off sugars for an extended period of time, you'll know that cravings grow stronger and stronger at first (but if you stick it out, eventually they'll weaken and disappear).

Chronic yo-yo dieters and drug addicts alike are prone to binging on their substance of choice during withdrawal recovery periods, when they're especially susceptible to relapse.[149] Many of us have been there: wolfing down a whole sleeve of cookies after dutifully sticking to a diet all week. But when we give in to these temptations, we only further the cycle of addiction and make it harder to quit for good. The impulse to relapse and binge on sugars comes from the desire to avoid the unpleasant symptoms of withdrawal, yet it's only by allowing the body time to re-balance its chemistry that we'll be able to make it through to the other side.

We all know how hard it can be to break habits. Quitting is never a one-step solution, but an ongoing process; just think of former cigarette smokers or alcoholics who might still feel temptation after years of kicking the habit. It's easy to fall off the wagon when we live in a world of constant enticement — and sugar, as we know, is everywhere.

We'll talk more about addiction and learning how to quit in the coming chapters. But first, I want to look at the toxic mental states, so common in modern American life, that often drive us to eat sugar in the first place: stress and depression.

CHAPTER 17

Fight, Flight, or Fat

S TRESS ISN'T WHAT IT USED TO BE. Our ancestors of the prehistoric age would have experienced stress in large, acute ways: defending themselves from wild animals, for example, or warring with other human clans for territory. Stressors were a thing to be confronted and conquered; generally speaking, you either won or lost, and then you could forget about that stress until the next problem came along.

When we perceive an immediate threat — whether it's a charging mastodon or a near-miss car accident — our bodies react with the well-known "fight-or-flight" response, where we instantaneously assess whether we ought to try to overcome it with a fight or if it's best to remove ourselves as quickly as possible. The body's internal reactions happen automatically. The kidneys secrete a wave of the hormone epinephrine (or as it's more commonly known, adrenaline) that sharpens our senses, increases our heart rate, and heightens our awareness: an "adrenaline rush."

But there's another reaction going on, too. Epinephrine triggers another hormone, cortisol. Cortisol reports directly to the liver, which, as we know from previous chapters, both stores extra glucose energy from food and is able to create energy from that glucose between meals. Cortisol alerts the liver that the body is in crisis, that it may need extra energy to fight or flee. All other digestive processes are temporarily halted, with efforts devoted exclusively to the production of extra glucose energy to be sent out to the body — just in case we need to flee *really* quickly.

In those situations that require split-second decisions or super-human strength (we've all heard the stories about a mother lifting a car to save her children, right?), the extra energy produced through cortisol can be a life-saver.

But in most cases today, stress is an entirely different beast. Day in and day out, many of us are plagued by the constant strains of work demands, social relationships, financial concerns, and the general stress from living in a fast-paced world. This kind of chronic, prolonged stress still triggers the same evolutionary hormone systems that saved us from wild animal stampedes thousands of years ago. But they're not likely to save us from an overflowing inbox.

When stress is constant and unceasing, cortisol stays on the job, too, continuously sending messages to the body to over-produce glucose energy and pump it into the bloodstream, where blood glucose levels and insulin levels stay elevated accordingly. If stress is physical — if we actually have to run away or lift up a car to save our children — the extra glucose energy gets expended and burned off. But what if we're just sitting behind a desk all day? Little of that extra energy actually gets used up; instead, the body has to find places to re-store it, usually as fat.

Because cortisol affects glucose, and because glucose affects insulin, chronic stress is also a dangerous risk factor for the development of aspects of metabolic syndrome, from diabetes, hypertension, and obesity to the more life-threatening complications of heart disease.[150] We've long known that too much stress can be harmful to the body, but looking at the exact internal mechanisms may give us surprising reasons why.

Stress tends to affect people's eating patterns in one of two ways: eating too little or eating too much. As the digestive process slows and cortisol commands the liver to produce extra glucose energy under stress, we may not feel hungry for unusually long periods of time. On the other hand, because so

140

much reserved food is being converted into energy, the body may cry out suddenly and acutely to replenish the emergency supplies as quickly and efficiently as possible. Refined sugars, as we know, are an abundant source of glucose energy that can be delivered to the body very rapidly. So when the body requires more supplies, it will naturally send us into cravings for energy-dense foods. Higher levels of chronic life stress are greatly associated with higher preferences for foods with a lot of sugar, since they're often the quickest way to restock glucose supplies.[151] But of course, when we're stressed from sitting in traffic all morning, that energy doesn't actually get used up or go anywhere (except maybe our love handles).

Stress mechanisms are really promoting the production of excess body fat from two angles: they encourage the consumption of more calories from energy-dense foods, and they encourage the storage of unused energy as fat. (Unsurprisingly, exercise is a great stress reliever because it gives all that extra glucose energy a purpose.) Stress problems and weight problems tend to be related in the United States. Overweight people tend to report higher levels of stress than others, but it might be more accurate to say that stressed-out people tend to gain more weight.[152]

Our internal stress response is so powerful that it can overwhelm even the best of our intentions: people who are dieting by restricting their calories (more than 100 million Americans on any given day) are much more likely to break their diets and over-eat during times of stress. They're also likely to overeat more than non-dieters.[153] And let's face it: dieting is stressful in and of itself. People who are overweight and stressed are more likely to make attempts at developing healthier eating habits, but they're also more likely to fail.[154] With our stress response systems set up the way they are, and faced with unrelenting pressure at work, home, and in between, who can blame them? Chronic stress sets us up for failure, especially when fat-fueling sugars are readily available at every turn.

I believe that it's no coincidence that our society is becoming increasingly burdened with stress, obesity, and heart disease all at once. And it's no accident either that refined sugars are as abundant and popular as they are. We crave them — physically, mentally, and, well, hungrily. We've come to depend on sugars to fuel us through times of stress (which, for some of us, is all the time). It's not just a separate health issue; stress is an integral factor in the perpetuation of our sugar-soaked society, one that we'll have to confront if we want to conquer our sugar addictions. There are healthy ways to deal with stress, and there are sugary ways to deal with stress. But it may be that stress is the problem itself.

CHAPTER 18

The Depression Diet

AMERICA IS A SAD COUNTRY — and I mean that quite literally. Rates of depression are forever climbing in the modern age. More than one in ten Americans today over the age of 12 are prescribed some kind of antidepressant medication, and it's assumed that many more experience depression without ever seeking medical or professional help. About $10 billion dollars are spent on antidepressants every year, making them the second-most highly prescribed drug in the nation (right after cholesterol-lowering statins, which we talked about in previous chapters).[155]

The majority of antidepressant medications on the market are what's called selective serotonin reuptake inhibitors, or SSRIs, which work by recycling supplies of serotonin, a neurotransmitter in the brain. Serotonin plays a key role in the regulation of our moods, sleep patterns, and appetites; a serotonin deficiency is thought to be one of the principal neurological factors behind major depressive disorder.

SSRI drugs work by helping the serotonin already present in the brain trigger multiple sensors, so that the mood-elevating chemicals can have a greater effect. They're largely successful in treating many people with depression, but we still have to wonder: What could make an entire 10% of the population serotonin-deficient to begin with?

The body cannot produce serotonin on its own; it's developed inside our bodies using ingredients from the foods we eat. One of serotonin's key components is an amino acid called tryptophan — famously abundant in Thanksgiving turkey, but also plentiful in all sorts of foods: nuts, meat, legumes, beans, seeds, eggs, leafy greens, and more. Contrary to popular belief, tryptophan doesn't make you drowsy (but all the sugar most of us eat on Thanksgiving probably does). Tryptophan is one of nine "essential" amino acids the body needs, meaning it has to come from outside sources (i.e., the foods we eat).

The amount of serotonin in our brains is therefore limited by the amount of tryptophan the body has to work with. It only makes sense that the more tryptophan-rich foods we consume, the higher the potential levels of serotonin available to the brain.[156]

For various reasons, tryptophan isn't something that can be packed into a pill (purified tryptophan supplements *do* exist, but they've been linked to outbreaks of a potentially fatal neurological condition).

The link between diet and depression hasn't been studied extensively. But cross-country comparative studies have linked higher rates of average tryptophan consumption with lower rates of suicides[157]; conversely, there appears to be a positive correlation between national rates of refined sugar consumption and rates of depression.[158]

Given the wide variety of cultural habits between countries, there could be a lot of explanations for these correlations that don't necessarily have to do with sugar. But one thing's for sure: the more daily calorie space we give to foods that are low in nutrients and high in sugars — like so many processed foods — the less likely we are to be consuming healthy, whole foods containing the necessary amounts of tryptophan to produce adequate serotonin for the brain. We're shortchanging ourselves, opting for the quick high of endorphin- and dopamine-triggering sugars instead of the stability and balance that can come from tryptophan-containing foods.

In fact, sugar might actually damage our ability to form serotonin. Amino acids like tryptophan are made available to the rest of the body through the liver, which, as we know, can be severely affected by the overconsumption of refined sugars. Alcohol abuse — which, metabolically speaking, looks very similar to sugar abuse — has been shown to decrease the bioavailability of tryptophan by as much as 26%.[159] Our nutrient-poor, sugar-rich diets may not only be shortening our lives and widening our waistlines; they might be making us miserable in the process.

Sugar's ability to stimulate the dopamine and endorphin systems of the brain might briefly counteract the detrimental effects of serotonin deprivation, but it won't change the underlying problem. Relying on the quick, artificial fixes of hormone bursts that come from sugar can snowball into patterns of addiction, only making things worse in the long run. The more sugar we eat, the less chance we have of maintaining a healthy, happy mood. We depend on foods to regulate so many functions of our bodies and minds; it should never just be about keeping our bellies as full as possible.

Serotonin, dopamine, endorphins, and cortisol all link in with a vicious cycle of sugar consumption. The more we try to medicate ourselves with sugar, the deeper we're pulled into habitual patterns of eating that can wreak havoc with our bodies and our brains alike. Sugar only digs us deeper into the rut it put us into in the first place.

CHAPTER 19

The Big Question

S UGAR'S ABILITY TO MANIPULATE the neural pathways that control our moods, appetites, sleep patterns, and behaviors brings us back to that big question: Can it really be addictive?

Many of us will admit to liking, wanting, or even needing sugar at certain times of the day — dessert cravings, afternoon sodas, etc. — but are we willing to own up to a full-fledged admission of addiction? And if we are addicted, is it a cause for serious concern? Are sugars really as perilous as drugs, alcohol, or nicotine?

Let's look at what we know. An addiction becomes a problem when the desire or need for a substance begins to interfere with our daily lives: our ability to work, our family or social relationships, our health, and our state of mind. A sugar-abuse dependency problem might sound exaggerated, but let's explore the question systematically. Start by asking yourself the following:

(1) Have you ever decided to stop eating sugars for a week or so, but only lasted for a couple of days?

(2) Do you eat a lot of sugars when you are disappointed, under pressure, or have had a quarrel with someone?

(3) Do you ever feel guilty after eating sugar?

(4)   Do you envy people who can easily eat sugars in moderation or without gaining weight?

(5)   Have you ever been unable to stop eating sugars, even when you weren't hungry?

(6)   Do you have to have sugars at a certain time every day (with morning coffee, evening dessert, afternoon energy drink, etc.)?

(7)   Have you had physical problems connected with eating sugars (obesity, diabetes, tooth decay, etc.)?

(8)   Has a doctor ever recommended you cut back on your sugar intake?

Analyzing our sugar-consumption patterns with these kinds of questions might seem invasive or overwrought, but these are all actual assessment survey questions used by Alcoholics Anonymous and other abuse-screening agencies to gauge levels of addiction and dependency. Here, the word "alcohol" and its related terms have simply been changed to "sugar" and its related terms.

Today, we may see refined sugars as a benign aspect of everyday living and eating, but social perceptions can change over time. Cigarettes used to be endorsed by doctors. Morphine used to be marketed toward children. Alcoholism wasn't recognized as an addiction until the mid-1950s.

The more we learn about the ill effects of refined sugar — on our bodies, our brains, and our society as a whole — the more convincing the argument that we ought to take a moment to re-examine our relationship with the sweet stuff. Will our children's children look back on our sugar-filled eating habits and wonder: *What were they thinking?*

Consulting The Diagnostic Bible

No matter the substance, addiction manifests in remarkably predictable patterns. First comes a build-up of tolerance, as the brain and body become accustomed to regular use; then come increased dosages or frequency of use, followed by an eventual physical and psychological dependency, as we've discussed. Though these stages develop internally, addicts of all kinds also tend to display certain similar outward behaviors, as well.

The *Diagnostic and Statistical Manual of Mental Disorders* (DSM) of the American Psychiatric Association, the clinical bible of mental health professionals, outlines eleven common behavioral symptoms of substance-related and addictive disorders. A patient who matches two or three symptoms is usually considered to have a mild addiction; six or more indicates a severe substance-use disorder.

The breakdown of the DSM's criteria and how it applies to sugar is eye-opening. Let's take a hard look at each in turn.

(1) *Craving or a strong desire or urge to use a substance*

Granted, we may experience cravings for many different kinds of foods as our body's way of trying to tell us what we need nutritionally. Cravings for sugar are usually different. We don't crave the nutritive or energy-supplying properties of a soda — of which there are very little — we crave the taste itself. Subliminally, whether we can recognize it consciously or not, we crave the emotional high, the sensory satisfaction that comes from refined sugars that doesn't necessarily come from a carrot or hamburger. We crave sweets even when we're not hungry. The desire can haunt us for hours if left unsatisfied — and even then, it will linger or return very soon. It's not the food we're after; it's the sugar itself.

(2) *Tolerance or markedly increased amounts of the substance to achieve intoxication or desired effect or markedly diminished effect with continued use of the same amount of substance*

The neurological symptoms of substance addiction can be observed behaviorally. Gradually, our brains and our palates adapt to sugars, requiring more and more to feel the effects of a sugar high or even to taste a pleasant sweetness. This can happen on a personal level — eating two sweets when one used to be enough, for example, or increasing the amount of sugar in your coffee or tea — but it also happens on a macro level. Our serving sizes of soda have only increased through fast-food history, and the common consumption of sweets with, after, or between every meal indicates a greater cultural need for the taste of sugar. Research shows that, within the last fifty to one hundred years, even our fruits, vegetables, and grains have been selectively bred for higher sugar contents. For many people, our taste buds have become so accustomed to sugar that a food without any tastes bland; for a sweet to taste sweet today, it must be sweeter than ever before.

(3) *Use of a substance in larger amounts or over a longer period than was intended*

Again, the symptoms can develop personally and culturally. Perhaps we put off starting a sugar-free diet another day, or another week, or after one last sleeve of cookies. Perhaps we only meant to have a few bites of cake but ended up eating the whole thing. This type of indulgent, binge-like behavior tends to be unique to high-sugar foods. Other foods fill us up or cease to taste exciting, but sugar keeps stimulating our tongues and brains for more. And while sweet snacks might ostensibly market themselves as just that — snacks — too often, the high sugar content once reserved for treats and desserts has crept into our everyday, every-meal foods. Snacking itself has increased culturally, with more than 56% of Americans snacking three or more times per day, up from just 10% in the 1970s.[160] We as humans may have been using refined sugars for 1,000 years or more, but only in the last half-century have we become so dependent on it for our sustenance.

(4) *Frequent use of substances in situations in which it is physically hazardous*

(5) *Use of substances even though there is a persistent or recurring physical or psychological problem that is likely to have been caused or exacerbated by the substance*

For the more than one in three Americans who exhibit symptoms of metabolic syndrome — obesity, diabetes, hypertension, dyslipidemia, etc. — the damage from sugars is already done. Unfortunately, many people may not realize how directly soda or sugar consumption can increase the risk factors for heart disease, so they continue to eat, drink, and purchase high-sugar foods. But no one is immune to the physical and psychological perils of too much sugar. The occasional cupcake won't kill you — neither will an occasional glass of wine. It's the cumulative effects of a persistent, long-term overindulgence in sugars — or alcohol and drugs, for that matter — that will put anyone at risk for addiction. With sugar, that also means greater risk for obesity, heart disease, tooth decay, cancer, rapid aging, and psychological addiction.

> (6) *Failure to fulfill major role obligations at work, school, or home such as repeated absences or poor work performance related to substance use; substance-related absences, suspensions, or expulsions from school; neglect of children or household*

What if — like alcohol — sugar wasn't something we could consume at work? There's little reason to skip out on work or class to secure a sugar fix when there's most likely a vending machine down the hall. But could you last all day without a sugary snack, or might you be tempted to take a break and find a place where you could drink a Coke? And would you be distracted at your desk if you were craving a candy bar and couldn't have one all day?

Of course, we rarely have to go out of our way to satisfy a sugar craving. However, repeated snacking, by getting up from your desk and leaving to fulfill a craving multiple times a day, can have an effect on your work by constantly interrupting your train of thought. The effects of sugar might not be so acute as to immediately and drastically affect our work, school, or parenting obligations. But the long-term consequences of chronic sugar consumption can certainly lead to repeated absences — ill health, doctor's and/or hospital visits, not to mention an overall shortened life expectancy — and lost productivity. Moderately or extremely obese workers experience more health-related work limitations than other employees, especially when it comes to completing physical or timely tasks.[161] In all, the real value loss from every severely obese and metabolically unfit employee can amount to over $6,000 per year.[162]

(7) *Persistent desire or unsuccessful efforts to cut down or control substance abuse*

The diet and weight-loss industry is a $20 billion per year market. More than 100 million Americans are on a diet, yet we remain the world's fattest nation. No matter the strength of our willpower, it seems our self-control cracks under the pressure of sweets and sugars. We may want to break the habit — we may vow to cut back on sugars — but clearly it's much easier said than done.

(8) *Withdrawal symptoms or the use of certain substances to avoid withdrawal symptoms*

When cutting out sugars completely, people often report feeling tired and irritable; cravings for sweets can be intense. But even on a daily basis, many of us engage in withdrawal avoidance without thinking twice: when we hit a mid-day slump in the afternoon, we intuitively grab for sugar in the form of sweet snacks, sodas, or energy drinks.

Yes, they'll perk you up, but only because the body has become dependent on a constant influx of refined sugars to remain stable. Withdrawal can be a difficult and unpleasant experience; it might be easier to just keep on with sugar, but it only exacerbates our problems of dependency. After a complete and extensive detox from sugar, most people will be able to return to normal — or often, even better — functioning and alertness with far fewer cravings for sugar.

(9) *Continued use despite having persistent or recurrent social or interpersonal problems*

(10) *Reduction or abandonment of social, occupational, or recreational activities because of substance use*

In our discussion of the "depression diet," we saw how a cycle of self-medication with sugar can ultimately worsen depressive moods, which can lead to more social withdrawal and lethargy.

If we gain weight from sugar, we set ourselves up for more psychological and emotional problems. Despite the fact that a majority of Americans — two-thirds — are overweight, we still largely consider being overweight a result of personal failure, laziness, lack of willpower, etc. Overweight and obese people are stigmatized in work and school settings, public spaces, and by the media, which can lead to varying degrees of depression, stress, and social ostracism, regardless of a person's actual physical health and ability. In turn, these feelings can trigger emotional patterns of eating even more sugar, further fueling a vicious cycle.

(11) *Involvement in chronic behavior to obtain the substance, use the substance, or recover from its effects*

We're rarely more than an arm's reach away from sugar or sugar-containing foods, so we may not be entirely conscious of how many times a day we seek it out. If we start every morning with sweetened yogurt, orange juice, or ready-to-eat breakfast cereals, is it a harmless ritual or a chronic behavior? Is a daily soda with lunch or a nighttime sweet dessert borne out of a like, a want, or a need for sugar? If suddenly we were transported to a remote area with absolutely no refined sugars, how far would we go to satisfy our craving?

Unlike many addictions, sugar use is so pervasive that we often have to work harder to avoid the stuff than to consume it.

Tallying the Results

By the American Psychiatric Association's standards, a person need only exhibit two of any of those above symptoms to be considered a mild addict.[163]

When it comes to sugar, many Americans can no doubt relate to many more than two of these symptoms. It's not just a personal struggle; it's a nationwide cultural struggle. Even if we're not personally affected by sugar addiction and its many adverse health effects, we are affected by the maelstrom of national consequences: overcrowded hospitals, higher health-care premiums, a decreased and less efficient workforce — and surely friends and family members who suffer, too.

If the spread of obesity continues at the same rate as it has over the past several decades, virtually *all* American adults will be overweight or obese by 2048.[164] It's time we not only take a hard look at the effects of sugar-fueled obesity but also question the reasons why we have so continuously and repeatedly failed at nearly all efforts to cut back on our sugar consumption and our growing waistlines for so many decades.

Is this an issue of personal accountability, or is it an issue of mental health and psychological addiction? The sooner we face our sugar demons, the sooner we can take the steps to correct the health crisis that is crippling America and rapidly spreading throughout the world. Admitting we have a problem, as they say, is the first step toward recovery.

CHAPTER 20

The Case for Sugarism

IF HUMANS HAVE BEEN CONSUMING refined sugars for so long, a valid question is: Why has it only become such a problem now? Why has the scourge of obesity, diabetes, and heart disease escalated to perilous heights only within the past fifty years, even though sugar has been a staple of Americans since before the United States was a country itself? How can sugar be the culprit of modern disease when it's an ancient ingredient?

The answer is a matter of quantity. Just like it's possible to enjoy an occasional — possibly even daily — glass of wine or bottle of beer without any long-term ill effects, it's possible to consume and enjoy sugar in moderation without metabolic consequences. But too much of either, over too long a period of time, can produce toxic effects that damage the body and manipulate the brain.

Researchers generally cap the maximum amount of alcohol that can be consumed without causing toxicity at 50 grams per day, or about three and a half drinks. Dr. Robert H. Lustig, the pioneer in sugar and obesity research we mentioned earlier, argues that the maximum threshold of toxicity for fructose (the simple sugar that comprises one half of sucrose or 55% of high-fructose corn syrup) is the same level as alcohol — 50 grams per day.[165]

So for sugar to produce toxic effects, one would have to consume 100 grams or more of sugar every day, or more than 80 pounds every year. Currently, the average American consumes nearly 130 pounds of sugar every year, or 60% above toxic levels. We're well over the threshold, and have been since the boom in sugar consumption after World War II. The catch is that the effects aren't immediate; they accumulate over time from excess consumption, resulting in adult-onset obesity, diabetes, and heart disease only after years of abuse.

As we've seen, fructose metabolizes in the liver in remarkably similar ways to alcohol; abuse of either can amount to fatty liver disease, cirrhosis, and liver failure. And alcohol and sugar stimulate similar regions of the brain, including the dopamine and endorphin pathways that can instigate tolerance and addiction. Brain scans of people who exhibited traits of sugar addiction displayed neural activity in the same areas when shown pictures of a milkshake as alcoholics did when shown a picture of an alcoholic beverage.[166]

Addiction research across substances repeatedly shows that a tolerance to one substance will transfer to other substances, especially when substances activate the same regions of the brain, producing what's known as crossover addictions.[167] Heroin addicts can easily become hooked on other opiate drugs like methadone or morphine; amphetamine addicts might transfer to cocaine for its stimulation of dopamine. Addicts *of all* kinds frequently show preference for high-sugar, very sweet foods, which activate *both* opioid and dopamine pathways, just like their hard drugs of choice.[168]

Alcoholism and sugar addiction are so neurologically and biologically similar that they may be one and the same. Alcoholic men prefer beverages with a much higher sugar concentration than do non-alcoholics,[169] and even the children of alcoholics are found to be more susceptible to developing a greater sweet tooth than those of non-alcoholics.[170] Dr. Kathleen DesMaisons, an addictions counselor, found success treating recidivist alcoholics — men with a repeated history of drunk driving who had been previously unresponsive to other forms of treatment or therapy — simply by changing their diets, too. In additional to traditional addiction therapy methods, DesMaisons had her patients remove all sugars and refined white starches from their diets; by the end of the program, 92% of the once-incurable men had gotten clean and stayed sober.[171]

Sugar acts in alcohol's absence. Apparently, when alcoholics quit drinking but stay primed on sugary foods, the brain and body cannot re-acclimate to normal levels of hormonal activity. A craving for alcohol is assuaged by sugar, decreasing withdrawal symptoms and leaving the brain primed for more simple sugars in any form. Alcoholics who medicate with sugar become more prone to relapse or simply become addicted to sugar substances instead of alcoholic ones.

The silver lining in relating alcohol and sugar is that the similarities between the two allow us to use what we know about one to help treat the other, or both at the same time. Some studies suggest that family history is a very strong predictor of substance abuse; as much as 60% of one's chances of developing alcoholism are influenced by genetics, leaving only 40% up to environmental factors.[172]

That's not to say that the children of alcoholics or sugar addicts are predestined to become addicts themselves. But a greater awareness and consciousness of the risk factors and environmental triggers could save a lot of people from the grips of substance abuse and the metabolic problems of obesity, diabetes, and heart disease.

By comparison, the physical manifestations and consequences of sugar addiction are much less influenced by genetic determination; only 10% of variance in metabolic syndrome is due to hereditary predisposition. The difference suggests that the metabolic consequences of sugar such as obesity are a product of our minds — not our genes, appetites, or willpower (or lack thereof).

In this view, obesity isn't a product of sloth or gluttony, but of the manipulative powers of an addictive, toxic, and potentially lethal substance. Alcoholism is classified as a disease. On a biological level, it's the afflicted body driving the choice to drink, and a sugar addict suffers from the same sort of condition.

At the same time, addiction shouldn't be seen as an excuse for behavior. We can't simply throw our hands up in the air, blaming the foods in the store or sodas in the fridge for our sugar epidemic. Pointing fingers won't get us anywhere. In many rehabilitation programs, patients are taught that they are not necessarily to blame for their substance dependency, but at the same time they must take responsibility for and accept the consequences of their actions. When we consciously acknowledge the power that refined white crystals of sugar have over us, we can begin to take the initiative to change and to better hold ourselves accountable for our own actions.

Conquering our mental hang-ups over sugar will help us conquer the physical setbacks, leading us all to a healthier, happier future.

PART V:

Public Policy

Dealing with Sugar

CHAPTER 21

The Blame Game

WHEN IT COMES TO THE PERENNIAL QUESTION of "What's for dinner?" we have more possible answers than ever before. With more than 42,000 products in the average supermarket, it's difficult to know what to eat, or even *why* to eat: Do we eat to nourish and energize our bodies, or do we eat just for the taste of it? Do we eat out of hunger or cravings, or both?

More than anything, processed food is designed for maximum ease, comfort, affordability, palatability, and uniformity. Sugar is the magical ingredient that satisfies all of these needs. And refined sugar is not just convenient; it's cheaper than almost any other food ingredient. Sugar made from cane in Brazil acts the same as sugar made from beets in Minnesota, making for a reliable product that food manufacturers around the world can depend on to give their products a look, taste, and mouth feel that customers anywhere will recognize and enjoy. Sugar works simultaneously as a preservative, a structural component, and a flavor enhancer in many foods — not just the obvious sweets like candies and cookies, but also in the not-so-obvious like wheat bread and potato chips. Without sugar to bulk up and fortify our foods, we likely wouldn't *have* much food — at least not the kinds of things we've come to expect from our grocery aisles.

People like sugar. They like it so much that they will continue to eat it despite satiety, despite the known undesirable consequences like tooth decay, weight gain, and even acne. The food companies clearly know and recognize our penchant for sugar. The more a product has, the better it tastes and the more likely customers will be to enjoy it. Forget sex; *sugar* sells.

But at what point should the corporations making the majority of our foods be held responsible for the effects of their contents? Are companies knowingly exploiting our weakness for sugar, pumping it into their products to sell more goods despite the known health hazards? Or, on the other hand, are they simply giving us what we ask for?

The problem with addictive substances — like tobacco, alcohol, and sugar — is that there will *always* be a demand. For perfectly legal substances like sugar, this puts suppliers in a bind. Say one food manufacturer were to step up to the plate, admit that sugar is a harmful and toxic additive, and vow to discontinue its use in their products for the good of the consuming public. Some other, perhaps less noble, company would quickly be able to swoop in and fill the demand. Such is the free market society: companies only stand to lose profit by cutting sugar, even if it's the right thing to do. If sweeteners were banned or regulated, it's not too far-fetched to imagine bags of white crystal selling on the black market.

If the flow of supplies won't willingly stop, we'll have to take it upon ourselves to curb the demand. There are multitudes of reasons to attempt a societal shift away from our current sugar culture, not least of all for the sake of our own physical and mental health. It'll also be good for the nation at large: veteran senior officers of the U.S. Armed Forces have declared obesity a "threat to national security," as over 27% of young men and women eligible for service are "too fat to fight."[173]

It's clear that a change is needed. We need to tackle our sugar problems, and soon. But it's difficult to know where or how to start. Can we depend on ourselves and our neighbors to boycott sugar in the name of demanding healthier food choices? Can we count on food corporations to honestly develop and deliver better alternatives, or will we have to turn to government regulation and legislation to get a handle over our extreme usage? Whose responsibility is it to make the first move, and will it really lead to change?

Striking a balance is difficult because consumers undeniably ought to have a right to eat and drink as they please. No one really wants to be told what to do, least of all by the government. There's a fine line between private intrusion and public safety, however, because it's not like one soda will instantly kill you — but many sodas eventually can. It seems paradoxical at the moment for our government and tax dollars to provide health care coverage that treats sugar-induced diseases, such as type 2 diabetes, while simultaneously subsidizing the production of crops that can cause such afflictions in the first place, like sugarcane and corn for high-fructose syrup. It's paradoxical that we tell our children to make healthy choices and then flood their school cafeterias with sugary drinks and snacks.

Ultimately, I think we're going to have to choose between the health of the population and the free market reign of sugar. As long as sugar's there, we're all going to be tempted to eat it. We're going to need some help in the battle to resist. Ideally, the sugar crisis could be solved by equal cooperation and support from all sides: consumers, government, and the food industry itself. As individuals, we need to change our own habits and encourage the change in others. The government needs to provide better public education about the dangers of excessive sugar consumption and to support proper nutritional science over special interest politics. We need to see to it that our foods are clearly labeled and fairly marketed, and for that we will need the collective support of the food companies themselves to help foster a cultural shift to healthier eating practices with the offering of better products.

It all sounds like an ambitious agenda. But if we want to save our health, cutting down on sugars will be crucial. Prevention is a far better solution to solving chronic metabolic disease than any of the world's most impressive medical technologies. We can stop the symptoms before they start if we learn how to combat our sugar addiction.

By emphasizing preventive education, nutrition, and medicine, we could likely avoid nearly three million cases of diabetes, over nine million cases of heart disease, and three million cases of cancer, just within the next twenty years. We'd reduce the national costs of illness by 27% — well over $1 trillion — and improve our health, longevity, productivity, and quality of life along the way.[174]

To stop the epidemics of obesity and heart disease, we have to start where we have the most control: our own plates.

CHAPTER 22

Sugar Patch Kids

IN ORDER FOR PREVENTIVE HEALTH MEASURES to be effective, we have to be ready to intervene and educate early in life. With one in three children in the United States today already overweight or obese, we need to start educating our youth on nutrition and the dangers of excess sugar consumption earlier than ever — before it's too late.

Many schools already have nutritional education programs, but when the childhood obesity rate has tripled over the past thirty years, one has to wonder how effective they really are. Studies show that simply telling kids to eat right and exercise has no effect in preventing or reducing weight problems in school communities.[175] How can it, when temptations appear in every hallway vending machine and behind every lunch counter?

The contradictions between the "eat healthy" messages of nutritional education and the realities of food offerings in schools are enough to confuse kids at any age. Vending machines full of sodas, fruit juices, and sugary snacks are readily available in middle and high schools across the country — and that's just the beginning.

The National School Lunch Program was established after World War II as a national security measure: more than 16% of all voluntary military recruits had to be turned away during the war years because they were either too thin or malnourished to serve their country. By providing low-cost, ample nutrition to the youth of America, the government hoped to ensure the country's future safety and health. However, today our problem is quite the opposite. As we said, twenty-seven percent of young people aged 17-24 are too overweight to participate in military service, and our school lunches may again be a part of the problem.

It's not an issue that's gone completely unnoticed: the USDA has taken steps to regulate the content of school-provided lunches. However, recent guidelines and mandates have largely focused on reducing the fat and sodium content of foods, almost entirely ignoring added sugars.

The irony of the federal prescriptions isn't just that pizza is considered a vegetable; it's that the tomato sauce on the pizza — the "vegetable" component — typically contains an entire packet of sugar for every quarter cup serving. And lunches often come with both fruit juice *and* a choice of milk (70% of kids opt for the chocolate-flavored variety) — both of which contain as much sugar as a soda. Foods sold at school kiosks or in vending machines, as per government restrictions, can be as high as 35% sugar by weight.

Getting the Message

Schools aren't the only place our children receive mixed messages about proper nutrition. The food industry currently spends $1.8 billion every year on marketing towards children; that's $24 for every child in the country. The average American child watches thirteen or more television advertisements for food every day, most of which are for fast food, ready-to-eat-breakfast cereals, candy, snacks, and sugary drinks. Ninety-eight percent of child-targeted cereal advertisements are for products high in sugar; the annual budget for cereal companies' promotional tactics is three times as much as the entire budgets for advertising fruits, vegetables, and dairy products *combined.*[176]

There's a lot of money invested in convincing children — who typically have little purchasing power of their own — to want and like certain products. Companies wouldn't keep spending money on advertising if it wasn't effective, of course; once kids get into certain eating habits, they're likely to carry them through adulthood. That includes everything from patterns of obesity — overweight children are more likely to become severely obese in adulthood[177] — to brand loyalty: more than 58% of all "children's cereals" (i.e., high in sugar) purchased are consumed by adults.[178]

Very young children are extremely impressionable when it comes to visual advertisements; most under the age of eight can't discern the difference between paid commercials and the actual program they're watching; they don't understand that commercials are designed to promote and sell products rather than educate or inform; and they often don't make mental distinctions between fantasy and reality. A superhero mascot who gets his powers from chocolate-coated cereal seems convincing and even plausible to young children. Many kids believe that the kinds of foods marketed toward them — high-sugar snacks, drinks, and meals — are what they're supposed to be eating.[179] *No matter what we teach our kids in schools, marketing efforts that promote sugar as healthy, "cool," or energy-boosting undermine any real educational efforts or parent-led examples.*

For more than thirty years, consumer interest groups such as the Action for Children's Television, the Center for Science in the Public Interest, the Consumers Union, and the Committee on Children's Television have advocated in vain for governmental regulations on child-directed advertising — especially for food products. In the 1970s, petitions to curtail children's sugar advertising reached the Federal Trade Commission, which subsequently proposed a ban on high-sugar food advertisements to young children. In response, more than 60,000 pages of written comments were submitted by interested parties — mainly from large food companies — to block the ban, utilizing more than $16 million in political lobbying efforts. The *Washington Post* editorialized the move as "a preposterous intervention that would turn the FTC into a great national nanny;"[180] the resulting backlash was a great embarrassment for the agency. The government revoked the FTC's authority to monitor child-specific advertising, and funding for the agency was cut drastically for more than a decade afterwards.

Nevertheless, child-directed advertising remains a concern at a national level. Freedom of speech and free-market capitalism allow child-directed sugar marketing to continue, but a more recent 2011 report from members of the FTC, the Food and Drug Administration, the Centers for Disease Control and Prevention, and the Department of Agriculture called for food industries to voluntarily set limits on children's food advertising. The report proposed that products marketed toward children ought to contain significant amounts of the food groups endorsed and recommended by the *Dietary Guidelines for Americans* (fruits, vegetables, proteins, and whole grains), and ought to limit the amounts of sugar, saturated fat, or sodium in high-profile advertised items.

The report was a challenge to the industry to hold itself accountable for its own actions on merely a voluntary basis. Still, protests flooded in. Some food industry executives called the proposed restrictions "bizarre and unconscionable"[181] while others deemed them "an unhealthy federal intention and impulse to ban free speech."[182] On the other hand, the voluntary nature of the regulations offered an ostensibly noble public relations move for many food companies; those who chose to adhere to standards could promote themselves as cooperating with and endorsing governmental nutritional guidelines. The Children's Food and Beverage Advertising Initiative (CFBAI), formed in response to the appeals for advertising regulations, is a self-regulated coalition of seventeen of the nation's largest food product companies, including Coca-Cola, Pepsi, McDonald's, Burger King, Kellogg's, and Hershey's, that pledges to "promote healthier dietary choices" through advertising. Combined, these seventeen companies account for more than 80% of all child-targeted food advertisements, and their uniform guidelines hope to set industry standards for health consciousness and corporate responsibility.

However, the CFBAI's list of nutritional criteria and "healthier choice" foods will raise eyebrows. Among the products that make the cut for children's advertising are Yoplait Trix Cotton Candy yogurt (which contains 14 grams of sugar per four-ounce serving), Capri Sun 100% fruit juice (21 grams of sugar per a small six-ounce pouch — a higher concentration than most energy drinks), and Fruit Gusher Snacks (which are an incredible 40% sugar by weight). These are the kinds of products that food companies deem "healthy" options for kids, leaving one to wonder what's in their "unhealthy" products.

Shared Responsibility

Arguments against advertising and marketing regulations maintain that it's the responsibility of parents — not the government — to monitor children's viewing habits and to teach them about advertising and proper nutrition. But marketing extends well beyond the TV set: children are more interactive with more varied types of media than ever before, and companies continue to find innovative ways to engage youth and get them to interact with their brands. Cereal companies produce worlds of online games that promote their products; social media and celebrity endorsements enhance the "cool" factor of certain foods that appeal to kids and teens. Coca-Cola was the first page site on Facebook to reach 50 million fans, and it consistently ranks among the top ten most-"liked" pages.

Soft drinks, snack foods, fruit juices, and cereals don't just sell a product to children: they attempt to sell a lifestyle. No matter how much we control our own children's media exposure and education, we can't control all children. And most parents will agree that peer influence can be overwhelming; no one in the school cafeteria wants to trade candy-like fruit snacks for an apple. Brand imaging of high-sugar drinks and foods makes them appealing to kids because they're fun and familiar, even if we tell our kids to just say no.

We don't hand out cigarettes during anti-tobacco campaigns, yet we stuff our children with sugar-filled lunches and snacks even as we try to coach them in healthy eating habits. Since Congress banned television and radio advertisements for cigarettes in 1971, smoking has decreased by 50% in the United States. Sugar poses a greater and costlier public health threat than smoking: one in four deaths in America stem from heart disease; one in five from smoking.[183]

169

Cigarettes, too, were once regarded as cool, once used cartoon characters to promote their brands, even continuously rolled out fun, new, fruity flavors. Incredibly, they were once given out as free samples to kids on school playgrounds. We managed to put an end to all that, while still allowing people the freedom to smoke if they so choose. No matter how much we educate, tax, or discourage the use of tobacco, there will still be people who smoke. The same likely holds true for sugar. The most important tactic in reducing smoking, though, has been the re-imagining of the product, reversing years of psychological marketing and advertising tactics. Modern anti-tobacco advertisements are graphic depictions of the consequences of smoking: cancer, heart attacks, and loss of limbs included.

The same health risks are possible with sugar consumption. What if, instead of the playful polar bears from iconic Coca-Cola advertising, the bears were depicted how they'd actually turn out from a lifetime of soda consumption: obese, diabetic, and depressed? "The Real Bears," a 2012 cartoon short produced by the Centers for Science in the Public Interest, makes a poignant satire doing just that. [184]

Required health labels on packages of cigarettes inform consumers of the dangers of smoking; should bottles of soda warn of the links between high sugar consumption and obesity, diabetes, stroke, heart disease, cancer, Alzheimer's, and tooth decay?

Do we really want our children going cuckoo for Coca Puffs any more than we'd want them to walk a mile for a Camel? Early engagement in healthy decision-making can help shape a lifetime of good choices. Yet as much as we educate, it's hard to quit sugar — or tobacco, or any substance — when constant reminders haunt you at every corner.

In early 2014, the pharmacy chain CVS announced bold plans to discontinue sales of cigarettes in order to better provide a congruous promotion of health care services for its customers. Yet sodas and sugary snacks fill the aisles, and candy litters the checkout counter. As a society, we need to match our actions with our words and offer a more unified approach to combating obesity, diabetes, heart disease, and sugar addiction.

Food specialists at the United Nations are convinced that "junk food and sugary drinks are like tobacco and deserve to be treated in the same way... Right now, advertising and availability are so pervasive and unavoidable that in many places people cannot choose to exist in a healthy environment; we must give them that choice."[185]

Consumer rights work both ways: we can have the right to choose potentially harmful products at our own risk, but we should also have the right to be informed of the dangers of such products and maintain the capacity to avoid them if we so choose. Today, you cannot walk a single block in any American city without the lure of soda, candy, and sugar-coated snacks beckoning from shop windows. We don't need to eliminate sugars completely, but we need to reestablish a sense of normalcy in the American consumer marketplace: food should be made of food, not sugar. If we want our children to eat right and live healthy lives, we need to give them the education and environment to get there.

CHAPTER 23

The Real Costs of Food

I T'S IMPOSSIBLE TO TACKLE the connected issues of sugar, obesity, diabetes, heart disease, and the American food chain without also examining the complex issue of poverty in the United States. As counterintuitive as it seems, families and individuals with limited, unreliable, or inconsistent access to food are up to 50% more likely to suffer from obesity than financial- and food-stable people.[186] Metabolic syndrome, the cluster of diseases that often predicate heart disease, is more prevalent among lower socioeconomic classes[187]; counties in the U.S. with the highest rates of poverty also bear the highest rates of type 2 diabetes.[188]

Fifty years ago, obesity, diabetes, and other products of metabolic syndrome were viewed as diseases of affluence: a sign that one could afford to eat well and enjoy a sedentary lifestyle. In some less-economically developed countries, this pattern still holds true. But as the overall wealth of a nation increases, so too does its levels of obesity and lifestyle diseases, especially when Western dietary conventions, like soda companies and fast food chains, begin to appear or become more commonplace. *There are now more people in the world dying from the excesses of food than there are people dying of starvation.*[189]

The surface explanation for this paradoxical trend is that high-calorie, sugar-rich foods have become cheaper and more affordable than healthy foods or whole foods. But that's not really the whole story.

Calorie for calorie, it's true that high-sugar drinks, snack foods, and prepared meals are cheaper than whole grains, fruits, vegetables, and lean proteins. However, that assumes that all calories are created equally. As an oversimplified example, take Little Debbie Boston Crème Roll Snacks. One box, or six servings, costs just $1.99 and packs a seemingly incredible value of 1,620 calories — less than one-tenth of a cent per calorie. However, the same $1.99 can buy one dozen large eggs, which could also easily supply six servings, but only 840 calories. Are Little Debbie snacks really twice the bargain of eggs, or are some calories better than others? The eggs provide protein, vitamins, and minerals; the cake rolls provide little. Which ones are more likely to sustain a healthy lifestyle?

In many low-income homes, the vital difference between the eggs and the cake rolls is that the eggs require time and energy to cook and prepare, while the snacks can be eaten on the go or packed into a lunch. Time is a resource as valuable as money; without it, people are more likely to purchase and consume convenience and ready-made foods.[190] People who work long hours in low-paying jobs just to make ends meet are not as likely to have the time or energy to prepare home-cooked, wholesome meals for themselves or their children. Additionally, eggs — or fresh fruits and vegetables — may simply not be as available in low-income urban or rural areas, where supermarkets and grocery stores can be scarce. Convenience stores, gas stations, and corner markets may have the only food available for miles, most of which is liable to be packaged products that are high in sugar and low in nutrition.

What We're Subsidizing

Sugary foods and refined sugars themselves may be exceptionally cheap and plentiful, but how did they come to be so? For every one acre of American soil currently growing some kind of fruit or vegetable, there are 34 acres planted with corn. Most of this corn goes to secondary sources — the production of animal feed, ethanol, or high-fructose corn syrup — rather than feeding people directly. Growing corn is much more heavily incentivized by government farm policies than any other food product because it's the cheapest source of plentiful calories. However, high-fructose corn syrup calories don't contribute to the health of the country in the way that calories from broccoli, beans, or blueberries might. By reallocating government farm-subsidy money towards fruits and vegetables and away from second-hand crop corn, we could lower the costs of healthier food options to compete with cheap junk food.

The 2014 Farm Bill has made great beginning strides: funding for fruits, vegetables, and organic programs increased 50% percent from previous years, totaling $3 billion in support. But it still pales in comparison to the $23 billion reserved for traditional (i.e., corn, soy, and wheat) crop subsidies.

The Farm Bill also provides funding for the nation's largest food assistance program, the Supplemental Nutrition Assistance Program, or SNAP, formerly known as Food Stamps. In 2013, some 47 million Americans — one in six people — received some kind of assistance through SNAP, which subsidizes the costs of food for low-income or temporarily distressed families and individuals. There's more than $70 billion tied up in SNAP money every year — money that the government feeds directly to the companies whose items are purchased by beneficiaries. More than two billion dollars of SNAP money goes towards the purchase of sugar-sweetened beverages every year,[191] money that companies want to ensure stays flowing their way. In 2011, former New York City mayor Michael Bloomberg advocated to remove soda from the list of SNAP-eligible food choices as a means to combat obesity and diabetes among the city's poor. Forces from the American Beverage Association, the Snack Food Association, and the National Confectioners Association — three powerful lobbies with heavy interests in sugar products — attacked the proposal as an infringement on consumer rights and a pathway towards a slippery slope of regulatory aims that narrow participants' choices.

The lobbies were right about one thing: it's unfair to stigmatize, target, and dictate the food choices of lower-income individuals when people with higher disposable incomes are 14% more likely to purchase and consume sweets on a daily basis.[192] However, measures that restrict SNAP eligibility requirements don't bar people from purchasing sodas, fruit juices, or soft drinks: it simply prevents them from doing so with government-subsidized dollars. SNAP beneficiaries purchase 43% more sugar-sweetened beverages than people of similar socioeconomic status without benefits — though they're no more or less likely to be overweight than the general population.[193] The prohibition of soft drink purchases with SNAP money would send a powerful message to all people that the government and the USDA, the bureau in charge of the program, do not view sugar-sweetened beverages as a nutritive food source. Whether the changes would lead to changes in the general purchasing habits of consumers, SNAP members or not, is less clear.

Rather than policing purchases at the checkout line, the SNAP program could encourage and incentivize the purchase and consumption of healthy food choices. An experimental trial that offered a 30% further subsidization of fresh fruits and vegetables within SNAP saw a 25% increase in purchases of such foods; direct cash vouchers that could only be used on fruits and vegetables in the Women, Infants, and Children (WIC) food subsidy program had similar effects.[194] Increasingly, certain states will also double the purchasing power of SNAP money when used at local farmers' markets, a move that benefits both low-income beneficiaries and local economies as well.

A Cheaper Solution

There is a cultural myth that cheap, sugar-laden, pre-packaged foods are the only way to sustain a diet when living on a restricted budget: people who must afford food exclusively through SNAP often live on $4.50 a day. However, a meta-analysis of food costs across the country found that the actual cost of the healthiest type of diet — one rich in fruits, vegetables, and lean proteins — and the least healthy kind — one full of pre-packaged foods and refined sugars and grains — differ by only about $1.50 per day.[195] Such a small margin, which surprised even the authors of the study, could be balanced in a number of ways: a mere $0.25 wage increase in full-time employment wages would cover the difference, as could a small but significant redistribution of government-supplied farm subsidies that lower the cost of healthy food itself. Even supplying the extra costs through SNAP — a total figure of nearly $26 billion per year — pales in comparison to the $147 billion currently spent on the medical costs of obesity annually.

Money alone cannot break the ties that bind poverty and malnutrition. We need to eradicate the assumption that healthy eating is more expensive — a view that benefits and is perpetuated by food companies themselves.

Low-income communities have a higher density of public advertisements for soft drinks and fast food than do more affluent communities,[196] and minority youth are exposed to twice the amount of advertisements for high-sugar drinks.[197] Marketing tactics that target the poor foster the idea that high-sugar foods and drinks are the only available, affordable, or satisfying options when living on a restricted income — a mindset that doesn't have to necessarily become a reality.

If we start putting our money where our mouth is on a federal level, we can support healthy buying options in our stores, healthy growing options for our farmers, and healthy eating options for all Americans.

CHAPTER 24

A Call for Action

AS LONG AS THERE IS REFINED SUGAR AROUND, there will be someone who wants to eat it — no matter the cost. Hundreds of years ago, people were willing to spend more than a day's earnings to purchase just a small amount of it. Millions of human lives have been wasted in slave labor among the sugar plantations. Wars have been won or lost in sugar's name. Today, we eat sugar to excess, even when it's poisoning us, leading to obesity and all of the other related diseases.

Without legal regulations or limitations, there will always be a way to make a buck off of sugar. We can't necessarily blame the Big Food companies for wanting to profit off our desires and addictions; if they don't do it, someone else will. For example, if General Mills were to take a moral stand against sugar and pull all of its highly sweetened cereals off the market — the Lucky Charms, the Trix, the Cinnamon Toast Crunch — they would only hurt themselves. Other brands' similar products would easily fill in the consumer gap left behind. Unless there is a uniform standard that holds all cereal companies, all soda companies, all snack and food companies accountable for their products, a free market economy will ensure that as long as there is someone to buy the product, it will stay on their shelves.

Efforts of intra-industry self-regulation so far have proven ineffective. Despite highly publicized pledges to reduce the sales of soft drinks in schools, to limit child-directed advertising of unhealthy food choices, and to provide clear and intelligible labels on food packaging, very little real change has happened. Sports drinks, fruit juices, and chocolate milk are prominent in every school cafeteria; children are witness to more food advertising than ever via the Internet; and cereals that contain more sugar than a glazed doughnut are stamped with a "Smart Choices" food label.[198] Our sugar consumption, obesity rates, and fatalities from heart disease are as high as ever.

The stalemate bears critical resemblance to the tobacco industry in the latter 20th century. Self-regulatory efforts saw little to no improvement in the public health crisis of smoking; it took governmental intervention to implement the changes that have since reduced cigarette use in the United States by 50%. The turning point came with evidence that Big Tobacco companies were aware of the health hazards, the dangers, and the addictive properties of their products — and continued to market them anyway. Can the same be said of Big Food or Big Sugar?

Again, we're not talking about outright prohibition. Responsible consumption is possible, but when it comes to addictive substances like sugar, it's irresponsible for the government to allow public indulgence to run rampant when the costs to society are so high. In order to properly regulate and raise public awareness about the ill effects of excessive sugar consumption, we can look at programs already in use for still-legal-but-regulated substances, like tobacco and alcohol, to figure out how to tame America's sugar beast.

Alcohol and tobacco products both carry warning labels that recognize a public consensus that ill abuse of these substances can bring permanent, lasting damage. And the situation is comparable: it's not one beer, one cigarette, or one soda that puts you at risk for disease and addiction; it's the long-term pattern of consumption. The difference with sugar, though, is that it's so widely pervasive in our food supply, it's difficult to know where to draw the line. Salad dressings containing sugar might not necessarily need to carry a warning label — although they should clearly indicate how much and what kinds of sugars are added — but products that are, for example, more than 25% sugar by weight ought to inform consumers of the risks and dangers of over-consumption; then, people can make informed decisions about whether or not to purchase and consume such products.

Food labeling practices in general need to be more specific about sugar content. Labels should differentiate not only between intrinsic and added sugars, but also between different types of sugars that can act very differently in the body. Of that fruit-flavored yogurt, how much sugar is from milk lactose? How much from the natural sugars of the fruit? How much extra sugar has been added for flavor? Is it fructose or glucose? Fanciful names that try to mask sugar for what it is need to be elucidated. Recently, the FDA declared the use of the term "evaporated cane juice" as another name for sugar as "false and misleading... [the] term falsely suggests that sweeteners are juice... [and] fail to reveal the basic nature of the food and its characterizing properties."[199]

It's time to take sugar for what it is, and allow consumers the right to know what's being poured into their foods.

Small Tax, Big Effect

Alcohol and tobacco are also taxed heavily by local, state, and federal governments. In 1991, the national average price for a pack of cigarettes was $1.67 (or just over $3 in current inflation-adjusted money). Today, the same pack can cost $12 or more in certain areas of the country. If part of the appeal of high-sugar drinks and snacks is that they're so cheap, would a "sin tax" on unhealthy products help curb their consumption?

In fact, many states already have minor excise taxes on certain products like soft drinks, candies, and chewing gum. They're often as little as a penny-per-ounce — negligible amounts when it comes to deterring consumer purchases, but enough to generate billions of dollars of government revenue every year. If the average soft drink costs $1.50, how much would prices need to increase in order to deter consumption? Fifty percent? One hundred percent? Taxing high-sugar foods would greatly affect the prices of hundreds of items in the average supermarket, furthering the risk of pricing low-income people out of food's reach. However, if the government re-invested the revenue generated from sugar taxes into further subsidizing the farming of healthy food and nutritional assistance programs, we could make better nutrition more available to everyone.

Money from taxes could also be implemented to further obesity- and disease-prevention programs in our schools. High-schoolers today may know how to invert fractions or identify iambic pentameter, but too often they don't know how to prepare a meal using whole, fresh ingredients. Cooking and gardening is part math, part chemistry, part environmental science, and part hands-on experimentation. Since the advent of convenience foods, the art of cooking once passed down from generation to generation has been increasingly forgotten; we can't expect children's parents to teach them how to eat properly if two-thirds of the adult population is overweight and lacking basic knowledge of nutrition to begin with. Prevention means not only teaching kids how to avoid unhealthy habits, but giving them the tools to engage in healthy ones.

Tobacco and alcohol are also limited in their availability and visibility in ways that sugar is decidedly not. Candies, sodas, and sweets are prominently displayed at every cash register in every store. Tobacco and alcohol have age-restriction limits for purchases; while requiring proof of ID to buy a Coca-Cola may sound heavy-handed, teenage boys are by far the highest consumer demographic for soft drinks and foods with high amounts of added sugar. Patterns of consumption — and addiction — start early.

Short of depriving children of candy altogether, we simply need to make sugar less instantly available: on the walk home from school or to a friend's house, while waiting in line at the check-out, or around every hallway corner in every vending machine for a cheap, cheap price. Most states prohibit the sale of high alcohol-content drinks in regular stores, relegating them to specific liquor-only stores with prescribed sales regulations and hours. While we may not want a sugar-only store, we need to take sugar out of the line of sight where it plays to our addictions and impulsive behaviors. Put it behind the counter instead of in front. Limit the sales of sodas within the vicinity of schools. Take familiar cartoon characters off boxes of high-sugar, low-nutrient cereals and snacks, which can greatly influence children's preferences.[200] Get sugar out of sight and show the dangers at point of sale, and it will be easier for us to get it out of mind.

The challenges of food regulation are unique in that we need food to live, but we don't need cigarettes or beer. We don't need sugar, either. Sugar is not a food: it cannot sustain life, it does not provide ample nutrition, and in large doses it can be a toxin. We can learn to live without sugar; when we do, the food companies will have no choice but to follow our lead.

Our foods should promote health and longevity, not addiction and disease. We all want to be a part of the solution, not the problem. Sugar's allure has held us captive for too long. It's time to break free of our candy-coated chains and save ourselves from becoming lifelong suckers for sugar.

CHAPTER 25

Quitting

THE SIMPLEST THING WE as a nation could do to cut back on our sugar consumption would be to stop drinking sweetened beverages. That includes not just soda but also fruit juice, sweet tea, energy drinks, sweetened coffee beverages, and sports drinks. Liquids, believe it or not, contribute more to our daily calorie intake than any other food group. But less surprisingly, most of the calories in those drinks come directly from added refined sugars.

Sixteen percent of the average American's daily calories come from added sugars — roughly 320 calories, if you're on a 2,000-calorie diet. Of those sugars, 36% (115.2 calories) come from sodas and energy drinks; 10.5% (33.6 calories) come from fruit juice; and 3.5% (11.2 calories) come from tea drinks.[201] Altogether, that's 50% of our added sugar consumption, just from beverages alone. Every day, 160 empty calories per person are sourced from drinks, which add up to 58,400 every year; that's the equivalent of nearly seventeen pounds of body weight! By just dropping those liquid calories from our national diet, total consumption of sugars in the U.S. would be cut in *half*, lowering us to rates that haven't been seen since before World War II.

If you do only one thing to cut back on sugar consumption, do this: *Drink more water.* You can add wedges of lemon or lime if you don't like the taste.

You can try infusing fresh fruit or herbs for a little pizzazz. You can even keep your tea, your coffee, and your milk. Just don't add sugar.

It's not to say that sweet drinks are the only culprits. Refined sugars have become so ingrained in our eating culture that we're not always consciously aware of ingesting them: skipping the soda and candy aisle at the grocery store is obvious, but there are hidden sugars in so many packaged foods, even those that try to hide under the guise of healthy products or brand names. Yogurt is a classic example: a 5.3 ounce container of plain Chobani Greek Yogurt contains only 4 grams of sugar, presumably all of which are from the harmless milk sugar, lactose (half glucose, half galactose). Meanwhile, the same size yogurt in black cherry flavor packs in a whopping 21 grams of sugar — partly from the lactose, but also from the pureed fruit (which may lack the fiber and nutrition of whole fruits), evaporated cane juice (simply another name for table sugar), and fruit juice concentrate (again, no fiber — just sugars). With 17 grams of added sugars — sugars which are not intrinsic to the food itself, in the way that lactose is to yogurt — a woman who starts her day with black cherry yogurt (and with good intentions, since there's much popular conception that Greek yogurt is healthy for you) has already consumed over two-thirds of the American Heart Association's recommended maximum allotment of 25 grams of added sugars per day, before breakfast is even over. A woman who has plain yogurt, on the other hand, hasn't consumed any added sugars.

Current food labels don't tell us which sugars are which — whether they're added or intrinsic, whether they're from glucose, fructose, lactose, sucrose, etc. The American Heart Association itself has conceded, "To figure out if a packaged food contains added sugars, and how much, you have to be a bit of a detective."[202] In fact, at the time of this writing, nowhere on Chobani's ingredients list is there even a mention of the word "sugar" — but it's there; in three different forms, no less. Without a bit of math, close reading, and some mental reasoning, it's virtually impossible to tell exactly how much and what kinds of sugars are in our foods.

Unless we can persuade the government to enact changes in legal food labeling policies (more on that later), it's up to us, the consumers, to deduce what's in our foods through number-crunching, clever sleuthing, and some basic label literacy. Food companies hide sugars under all kinds of different names intended to sound either healthier or more mysterious: sugar, organic sugar, raw sugar, brown sugar, demerara, turbinado, muscovado, evaporated cane juice, dextrose, Florida crystals, beet sugar, castor sugar, crystalline fructose, sorghum syrup, grape sugar, refiner's syrup, date sugar, agave nectar, invert sugar, fruit juice, fruit juice concentrate, golden syrup, panocha... The list goes on. There might be plenty of code names for refined sugars, but they all act the same way in our bodies and our brains.

The abundance of terms can make it difficult to determine exactly how much sugar a product contains, or if indeed there's any at all. Current food labeling laws require that ingredients be listed by weight, from most to least. To avoid placing "sugar" as one of the top ingredients, companies might spread the total sugar content over several different varieties or names. For example, Nabisco Wheat Thins — supposedly savory, not sweet — list sugar, malt syrup, and invert sugar in their ingredients list for a total of 4 grams of sugar per 31 gram serving, or 13% sugars by weight. A jar of Bonne Maman Strawberry Preserves lists fruit as the first ingredient, followed by "sugar," "cane sugar," and "concentrated lemon juice" as the second, third, and fourth ingredients. There's no way of telling how much sugar these three "different" ingredients tally up to, or how it compares to the intrinsic sugar content of the actual fruit inside. It's quite possible that the three sugars combined would actually put it at the top of the ingredient list, outweighing the fruit content.

Clearly, the odds in the grocery market are stacked against us if we want to reduce or cut out our refined sugar consumption. But the first step in successfully cutting back on sugars is the simple awareness of our food environment. It takes some time, a developed sense, and some elementary math skills, but eventually picking up a food package to scan the label becomes an automatic habit. Better yet, avoid foods with packages or labels completely: whole foods like fruits, vegetables, and nuts are always a healthy choice, and can substantially satisfy cravings for sweets or snacks without overloading the body with refined or added sugars. Once you've learned to decode for sugar, it can be astounding to realize just how prevalent it truly is in the marketplace. Our culture isn't set up for a sugar-free diet; it's understandable if we all feel a little like an alcoholic in a liquor store.

Cold Turkey

When it comes to taking action, many people find it best to quit sugars all at once. But first, you have to prepare yourself. Learn what foods do or don't contain refined sugars, and gradually remove the ones that do from your house — taking care to be well stocked in foods without sugars. That way, you'll be well armed when cravings strike.

Prepare your house ahead of time: Buy plain yogurt or oatmeal, which might taste very bland at first to the sugar-accustomed palate, but try sweetening it with bits of whole fruit or raw honey (if you must use a sweetener, use raw — not pasteurized — honey, which is the most natural of all sweeteners and contains many intrinsic vitamins and minerals). Replace soft drinks with lemon water; opt for sugarless versions of peanut butter, mustard, salad dressings, or any other condiments you keep on hand.

Planning ahead and learning what foods have excessive added sugars is the most important aspect to successfully cutting out sugars. Guard yourself from temptations at home, at work, or even on the commute by staying stocked with snacks without added sugars, such as dried fruit or nuts. Build a support network — challenge family, friends, or co-workers to embark on a sugar-free challenge with you. Plan a one-week, ten-day, or month-long sugar cleanse — or have a contest to see who can hold out the longest.

Going cold turkey, in my experience, is the best way to ensure success. Remove sugars from your sights as much as you can, and give your body the time to re-adjust to a non-addictive way of eating.

The first 24-30 days will be the most difficult. There will be cravings. There will be fatigue, irritability, possibly even headaches or shakiness. There will be times when you want to give up. But trust me: the longer you hold out, the easier it will become. After the first two months up through the six-month mark, your body will start to recognize this as the new norm, but cravings will still be present and strong as you've likely had a lifelong history with elevated sugar consumption. From there through two years after "quitting" sugar, you will notice that cravings will be milder and continue to weaken and will occur at a lower frequency, eventually disappearing almost entirely. It's most important that you recognize that this is a process that will take twelve to twenty-four months to fully get control over, but it does get significantly easier as time passes and you establish new eating habits.

An important note, though, about going sugar-free. Artificial, non-caloric sweeteners like Splenda (sucralose), Equal (aspartame), or Sweet'n Low (saccharin) are not, as far as we know, appropriate substitutions for sugar. Not enough research has been done to determine their safety in human diets; some studies even suggest that their use leads to more weight gain than the use of regular sugars.[203] That's because the sweet taste of artificial sweeteners primes the body and the brain for an influx of sugars — but since the actual sugar never comes, the hormones that regulate hunger, digestion, and the reward pathway of eating go unabated, and cravings for more food and sweets can actually increase.

The point of eliminating refined sugars from our diets is to free ourselves from the perpetual cravings — not to trick our taste buds into thinking they're taking in something they're not.

Artificial sweeteners are chemicals that have been formulated in laboratories (often by accident) and then quickly rushed on to the market without proper study of their effects. Current food regulations by the FDA tend to assume that foods are safe for consumption until enough evidence accrues that they are unsafe. Without enough long-term, large-scale studies, we don't really know how harmless or harmful artificial sweeteners are, or what their effects on our bodies and brains might be in the long run. Instead of breaking bad habits, they perpetuate sugar-eating patterns, only using a false substitute. The safest way to kick the sugar habit is to eliminate the taste completely.

The sooner you can go sugar-free, the more things like plain yogurt and oatmeal with some fresh fruit will taste plenty sweet — I promise, because I've experienced it.

The Plan

Sugars are lurking everywhere in our stores and shelves, and by this point, you might be wondering: Well, what *can* I eat? I'm not here to promote any particular kind of diet. I'm here to get you to get rid of sugars. That's it. But I understand from personal experience how frustrating it can be to find a new way of eating and change your life after depending for so long on sugary foods like cereal for breakfast or soda to get through the day.

Planning and preparedness is key to staying off sugar. If you make smart decisions ahead of time, it'll be easier to stay on track and fight the cravings when they hit. Go for "whole" foods — ones that don't require going through a manufacturing plant — over processed ones. Reach for water instead of juice. Create meals that you will enjoy eating, and take the time to revel in the way real food nourishes your body, inside and out.

The personal choice to stop the vicious cycle of sugar consumption must first come from within. When we hold ourselves accountable for our purchases, diets, and actions, we can better control our health and well-being.

But mental resolve isn't always enough to overcome addiction: our culture is so saturated with sugar that temptations will lurk around every corner. We are not invincible, and we will likely slip into the comforts of sugar now and then. The goal is not perfection. This is not a diet to go on and off at will. This is about changing your lifestyle. It may not be 100% sugar-free, 100% of the time. Kicking sugar is about doing the best you can: learning how to better engage in conscious decisions about foods, understanding the consequences of your actions, and figuring out how your body can live up to its fullest potential. The more we moderate our sugar intake, the better our health will be.

A grassroots approach to combating the sugar epidemic may be the most effective way to implement overall change in our food system. As consumers, we hold purchasing power: the less sugar we buy, the less food companies will be able to profit off of sugar-enhanced products. Food corporations respond to consumer demands, so we have to tell them what we want — or don't want — through our voices and our actions.

Change that starts from the bottom can, with enough support, strike influence through to the very top.

Eat This, Not That: Practical Tips for Quitting Sugar

- Your Most Likely Culprits: Foods to Avoid
  - Sodas
  - Fruit Juice
  - Energy drinks and bars
  - Snack bars with 5 grams or more of sugar
  - Any candies
  - Jams/jellies
  - Syrups
  - Ready-to-eat breakfast cereal containing more than 2 grams of sugar per serving
  - Pancakes, waffles
  - Flavored yogurt
  - Breads with added sugar (check your labels)
  - Bottled salad dressings with more than 2 grams of sugar per serving
  - Ketchup and barbecue sauces
  - Peanut butter

- All Systems Go: Foods to Substitute Instead
  - Fruits and vegetables
  - Potatoes and all tubers
  - Wild rice with hull
  - Hummus, olive tapenade, tomato salsa
  - Fish, poultry, beef, lamb
  - Eggs
  - Butter
  - Whole-grain bread with no added sugar

- Plain, sugar-free oatmeal and cold cereals — top with fruit, nuts, and cinnamon
- Hot cereals: grits, cream of wheat, or quinoa — top with fruit, nuts, and cinnamon
- Plain yogurt — top with fruit, nuts, and cinnamon
- Water infused with lemon, lime, mint, or cucumber
- Coffee, tea (unsweetened)
- Low-fat milk/almond, soy, or rice milk (unsweetened)
- Dry red and white wine (but be mindful as many wines have residual sugar and some have juice concentrates added which contain substantial amounts of sugar)
- *Natural* peanut or other nut butters (with no added sugars)
- Raw nuts (almonds, cashews, walnuts, etc.) with dried fruits (raisins, dates, pineapple, etc.) with no added sugar
- Seeds: flaxseed, chia seed
- Olive oil and vinegar for salad dressing
- All herbs and spices
- Sugar-free dry rubs

- Ways to fight cravings
    - No artificial sweeteners
    - Remove temptations from sight and keep out of reach
    - Keep fresh nuts and dried fruits (no added sugar) on hand at home and work
    - Distract your taste buds: use cinnamon, nutmeg, vanilla extract on unsweetened foods
    - Distract yourself: go for a walk when cravings strike
    - Do not go grocery shopping when you are hungry
    - Roast vegetables to bring out their natural sweetness
    - Plan meals in advance and eat at regular times
    - Try new foods — ones that don't have any sugar! Different varieties of fruits, veggies, or grains can excite the taste buds
    - Build a support network: Have people to talk to when a craving strikes who can both help and hold you accountable
    - Find healthy ways to manage stress/emotions that may trigger sugar-eating

- o Reward yourself occasionally with a *high-quality* (not quantity!) treat such as "ice cream" made with 1 banana, ¾ cup unsweetened almond milk, ¼ cup milk, and 3/4 cup of ice cubes in a blender

Don't blame yourself if you slip now and then. It's not about perfection, but about overall reduction. Start fresh every day!

Additional Dietary Principles

Hopefully by now, you are convinced that sugar is a toxin and is integrally linked to all the diseases associated with metabolic syndrome: heart disease, diabetes, obesity, dementia, polycystic ovarian disease, some forms of cancer, fatty liver disease (etc). While this book is not intended to be a nutritional guide, I would be remiss not to highlight specific food groups and nutritional categories that can promote a longer, healthier, and higher quality of life. Modifications of these suggestions can be made to fit your specific needs or beliefs if one is gluten-sensitive or vegan. The overall goal is to decrease the added sugar (especially fructose) in our diet. What you need to replace these calories with is fiber, protein, and "good fats".

The choices I outline below adhere to certain principles:

(1) Food items with more grams of sugar than fiber are to be avoided.

(2) Become a sugar detective…there are more than 55 names for sugar and the food industry wants to hide this addictive toxin whenever and wherever it can.

(3) Don't be fooled by labels that claim "no sugar added", "all natural", or "organic". (Juice with no sugar added is from concentrate and has had the fiber removed).

(4) Fat is not your enemy. Sugar bound to fat (glycated) is your enemy.

Carbohydrates

Don't fall into the "no carb" trap. Fibrous carbohydrates like fruits and vegetables have numerous vitamins, minerals, and micronutrients. It's the processed/refined carbs that are to be avoided!

Grains

Grains are the seeds of grasses. Whole grains are unrefined (no milling). They are better sources of fiber and micronutrients. However, all grains increase our insulin levels. Refined grains have been milled to increase the shelf life. The fiber and nutrients have been removed. Enriched grains have had some of the nutrients added back. They are fortified but lack fiber and are still missing some key nutrients.

Protein

Protein is an important component of every cell in the body. It is a macronutrient and we need adequate amounts of it. Your body uses protein to build and repair tissues and to make enzymes, hormones, and other body chemicals. It is a building block of bones, muscle, cartilage, skin, and blood. Promoting lean muscle development is one of the ways we fight insulin resistance. Increasing bone density can decrease the risk of osteoporosis. Protein also lowers blood pressure and improves brain function. A diet rich in protein increases satiety and decreases hunger. The best sources of protein come from fish, grass fed beef, poultry, nuts, whole grains, eggs, dairy, and beans. Avoid the processed meats.

Fat

The removal of fat from our diet in the 1970s is one of the key catalysts that got us into this mess. The alleged correlation between fat and cholesterol consumption and higher cardiac risk is an absolute fallacy. It was the greatest health scam of the century. Fat is the preferred fuel of human metabolism. The brain needs cholesterol. The higher the cholesterol level the lower the incidence of dementia and other neurological diseases. Cholesterol helps brain synapses through myelin coating, serves as an antioxidant, and is the precursor to estrogen, testosterone, and vitamin D. It is a myth that all LDL is bad. (LDL transports cholesterol into the neuron where it is needed. Only when *sugar* attaches to LDL does it become "bad." It then becomes oxidized, rendering it dysfunctional. This is what leads to the increased risk of dementia and atherosclerosis).

Trans fats are the dangerous fats. They are found in candy, desserts, cakes, cookies, chips/crackers, and fried foods. They are to be avoided.

Saturated fats have unfairly been demonized in the past. Recent studies show saturated fats increase both HDL and LDL. (the increase in LDL is the large buoyant benign particles that are not harmful to the arteries). Seek out saturated fats in grass-fed meat; organic milk, butter, eggs and cheese; and coconut oil.

Polyunsaturated and monounsaturated fats are deemed the "good fats". Unlike trans fats, they protect the heart, manage moods, increase mental sharpness, decrease inflammation, improve the cells responsiveness to insulin, and repair damaged cells. In particular, Omega 3 fats are the coveted choice. They are abundant in certain fish, olives, avocado, walnuts, coconuts, flaxseed, chia seeds, organic eggs, and wild meat. (Omega 6 fats, on the other hand, are pro inflammatory and are found in processed foods and vegetable oils. You want a diet with the lowest Omega 6/Omega 3 ratios). Canola oil has been touted as a good fat but has high levels of erucic acid, which is associated with heart disease. Also, the seeds to make canola oil are genetically modified and heavily processed. Of note, polyunsaturated fats oxidize under high heat so cooking with these fats release free radicals into the body, increasing your risk for many diseases. This is why cooking with coconut oil is safer than cooking with olive oil.

Legumes

Legumes are peas, beans, lentils, peanuts, and soybean. They have a lot of carbohydrates but are also high in protein and fiber and are a good source of iron, magnesium, potassium, and calcium.

There is some controversy surrounding the legume soy; its heart and cancer related health claims have been challenged by numerous scientists. Soy beans are consumed as whole foods in the East. But in the U.S., most of the soybeans we consume have been highly processed. Nearly 90% of all soy products in the U.S. come from soybeans that have been genetically engineered. Eaten as certified organic whole foods, soy is rich in nutrients and minerals and may have a myriad of health benefits. Fermented versions of soy (tempeh, tofu, natto, and miso) are recommended.

PART VI:

Epilogue

CHAPTER 26

Concluding Remarks

FOR CENTURIES, INFECTIOUS DISEASES were the primary cause of death in humans. Bubonic Plague wiped out a third of Europe in the 14th century, and smallpox killed close to a half billion people as recently as the 1900s. But gradually, the discovery of antibiotics such as penicillin and, later, the development of vaccines changed all that.

Thanks to medical advances, most people would say that we're living much longer lives than our ancestors. And they would be wrong!

Let me explain. In the past, the biggest factor in life expectancy was infant and childhood survival rates. In England during the 1600s, for example, average life expectancy was only about 35 years, but that's largely because two-thirds of all children died before the age of four. In Colonial America, 40% of children failed to reach adulthood. In some societies, babies weren't even named until they reached their first birthday.

But once people survived beyond the age of five—beyond the hurdles of childbirth, wars, and childhood disease—their lifespans could be quite long. Benjamin Franklin lived to age 84 and President John Adams lived to 90 at a time when the average life expectancy was 40 years. What has not changed dramatically over the last several hundred years is our *maximum* lifespan. In fact, now that infant mortality in this country has essentially stabilized, we may in fact be living fewer years than our predecessors, when the net effect of medical availability and advances are factored in. The bottom line: I fear we are at a tipping point, where our children's generation may fail to reach the lifespan of their parents.

The reason is that we've been suckered! Maybe not intentionally, but nonetheless we've been fooled. And it's not the first time. As a society, we place our trust and faith in the medical healers of our time who use the current "scientific data." But as we've seen repeatedly, they're not always correct in their assumptions or deductions.

In the 1930s and '40s, smoking cigarettes was encouraged for the treatment of throat irritation. Doctors used to encourage their use and endorse certain brands. Cigarettes were prescribed to pregnant women and even given out for free on the schoolyard. Remember Virginia Slims and the promise they would help women lose weight? Cigarettes were even touted to "pick you up when you are low" and "calm you down when you are tense."

Eventually, of course, research changed our thinking and behavior. But not before real damage was done.

The same sort of thing happened in the 1970s with the call to reduce fat consumption as a supposed way to decrease cholesterol levels and heart disease. The advice seemed logical then, but we now know it was a mistake. The sugar we favored over healthy fat is killing us. And the food industry with government support is doing what the cigarette manufacturers have done for a long time: produce and market a substance that has been shown to cause disease.

There is no question in my mind—and I hope in yours now, too—that the overconsumption of sugar is responsible for the chronic medical disarray we find ourselves in today. Its consumption may prove to be the single greatest contributing factor to our current epidemic of chronic disease. We can continue to invent medicines (statins, antacids, antidepressants, etc.) at enormous cost to combat the problems brought on by this dietary *toxin*. Or we can prevent some of them by changing our diet.

Make the wrong choice and we will most certainly raise a generation of less healthy children whose lifespan is shorter than our own.

OK, it's easy to say. But I know there are obstacles to overcome. First and foremost, it's difficult to "choose wisely" when 80% of our food sources have sugar as a prominent ingredient. Its availability is overwhelming. From grocery store aisles to school vending machines to every food mart in between, sugar is constantly staring us in the face. When we add to that our own brain's reward center sending signals to seek sugar, and our bodies telling us we're in a constant state of hunger, we have a perfect storm—a trifecta of reasons why we fail to resist!

Yet I know from personal experience that the benefits of avoiding sugar and carbohydrates are real and long lasting. I shared my own experiences earlier, but I now have many patients in my practice who are seeing similar amazing results from avoiding added sugar. They have more energy and they are more positive. Those with high blood pressure, high fasting sugar and triglycerides, and "bad" cholesterol are seeing their numbers normalizing after cutting out sugar. My patients have been able to reduce or stop their anti-hypertensives, antacids, and insulin substitutes. These changes are irrespective of exercise, though exercising seems to speed the process (while bringing other benefits, of course).

So what can we do to fix the problem on a larger scale? While I wouldn't want a society where we'd need a "sugar black market" to make a birthday cake for our children, I do think substantial changes need to be made. The government could subsidize fruit and vegetable crops more in line with how it subsidizes corn crops, making healthier choices more available and affordable. The government could force the food industry to properly label products so the consumer doesn't have to be Sherlock Holmes when checking for the amount of hidden sugar. Adding warning labels to foods and drinks that have more than, say, 25% of their calories derived from sugar might make people think twice about their purchase, as they should. And because of the enormous cost to both quality of life and increased health insurance premiums from these products, let's tax them and use the money generated for nutritional education.

Adding warning labels that say, "Excess sugar consumption has been shown to be dangerous to one's health" would also be a powerful deterrent. Minimizing the endless stream of commercial advertisements that bombard our youth might limit the numbers of kids going "cuckoo for Cocoa Puffs." Educating our schoolchildren about proper nutrition and then actually offering these healthy food options in the cafeteria over the sugary alternatives would end the current mixed message we're sending our children.

We the consumer need to say "no" to sugary items so the food industry either hears our collective outcry or watches its stock prices plummet. And we need to continue to educate ourselves and others about the harmful effects of sugar while promoting healthier choices.

The negative effects of sugar on our health can take time to develop, but like the sand that fills an hourglass, every grain of sugar adds up, ultimately affecting our health and quality of life. Now that we finally have the knowledge, we have a real opportunity to make a change. We deserve better and our children deserve better. It's time to stop being suckered. Let's end this addiction to a toxin that has no nutritional benefits. What's at stake is the chance to live a longer, healthier, and more productive life—to the full extent that our telomeres intended.

We can do this. Change for a better future can happen one bite at a time!

Acknowledgments

The development of this book has changed my life and, in many respects, made me a better pediatrician. I, of course, couldn't have done it without the help and support of my own close network of friends, family, and working community.

I would like to thank, first and foremost, the outstanding efforts of Sandra Canosa and the crucial role she played in turning this "what-if" idea into a completed book. Her extensive research and literary know-how have given this work its immense quality and credibility.

I also must thank the people at Lawless Publishing, namely the founder Jeanne Lawless Mercier, whose guiding "quality of life principle" contains two key elements of this book: the food one eats, and the environment one creates to live in.

I extend my gratitude to Mark Liu for his editing and stylistic contributions; Connor Smith, a real foot soldier throughout the process, for his contributions to the layout and editing process; Samantha MacFall for her graphic design additions to the book; and Alek Santiago, whose efforts have never gone unnoticed.

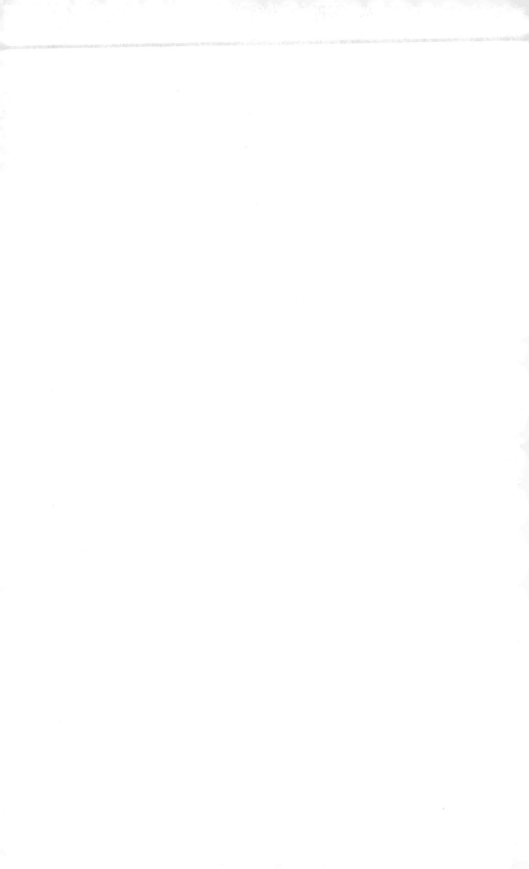

Glossary

Advanced Glycation End-Products (AGEs): a bonding of sugar to protein or lipids that renders them dysfunctional, leading to inflammation and a speeding up of the aging process; this plays a role in many degenerative diseases such as diabetes, atherosclerosis, and Alzheimer's disease

Atherosclerosis: the hardening of the inner artery walls by the deposition of plaque

Body Mass Index (BMI): one's Body Mass Index can be calculated by dividing weight in pounds by the square of height in inches and multiplying this number by 703 (if this number is in the range of 25-30 then one is considered overweight, greater than 30 classifies one as obese)

Cardiovascular Disease: an umbrella of heart disease that refers to narrowed or blocked blood vessels that can lead to heart attacks, chest pain (angina), or stroke

Caries: (or cavities): tooth decay

Cirrhosis: the late stage of scarring (fibrosis) of the liver; cirrhosis can be caused by alcohol, hepatitis B or C, and non-alcoholic liver disease (due to obesity, diabetes, hyperlipidemia, and hypertension, commonly known as metabolic syndrome)

Cortisol: the "stress hormone" best known for its involvement in the "fight or flight" response; produced by the adrenal gland, cortisol helps the body manage stress and utilize sugar and fat for energy; (chronically elevated levels of cortisol leads to elevated blood sugar levels, weight gain, immune system suppression, and high blood pressure)

De Novo Lipogenesis: the enzymatic pathway for converting dietary carbohydrate into fat for storage

Dopamine: our "feel good" hormone; it is a chemical neurotransmitter in the brain that sends messages between neurons, and helps control the brain's reward and pleasure centers

Dyslipidemia: an imbalance of fats (lipids) circulating in the bloodstream; specifically : elevated LDL known simply as the bad cholesterol, reduced HDL known simply as the good cholesterol, and elevated triglycerides

Endorphins: chemical neurotransmitters (our own endogenous morphine) that inhibit the transmission of pain signals and produce a feeling of euphoria similar to that produced by other opioids

Fatty Liver Disease: the accumulation of fat in the liver that results in inflammation and scarring; two main types: alcoholic liver disease (ALD) and nonalcoholic fatty liver disease(NAFLD) caused primarily by metabolic syndrome

Free Radicals: any molecule that has a single unpaired electron; they are unstable scavengers that steal an electron from a neighboring molecule rendering it dysfunctional, and are thought to be involved in the process of aging

Fructose: a monosaccharide that combines with glucose to form sucrose (sugar) and high fructose corn syrup; it occurs naturally in fruit, honey, berries and root vegetables; commercially it is derived from sugar cane, sugar beets, and corn

Galactose: the milk sugar; when combined with glucose, it forms a larger sugar called lactose

Glucose: the baseline sugar, this monosaccharide combines with fructose to make sugar and with galactose to make lactose (milk sugar); starches are just chains of glucose

Glycogen: a stored form of glucose chains that can be rapidly mobilized from the liver and muscle when available food energy is low

Heart Disease: see cardiovascular disease

High-Density Lipoproteins (HDL): lipoprotein molecules that transport lipids such as cholesterol and triglycerides away from artery walls back to the liver, thus decreasing atherosclerosis

Hypertension: high blood pressure

Hyperinsulinemia: excessive production of insulin

Insulin: the "storage hormone" produced by the beta cells of the pancreas that allows blood glucose to enter the cells and be used for energy; if your body doesn't produce enough insulin or your cells are resistant to the effects of insulin, high blood sugar (hyperglycemia) develops

Lactose: a sugar present in milk made up of two smaller sugars, glucose and galactose

Leptin: the "I'm full hormone" made by fat cells that tells the brain to stop consuming food; obese people make lots of leptin but the brain begins to "ignore" it; leptin resistance is the leading cause of fat gain as the brain erroneously thinks the body is starving

Low-Density Lipoproteins (LDL): lipoprotein molecules that transport lipids into the arterial walls resulting in atherosclerosis, heart attacks, and strokes

Metabolic Syndrome: a cluster of conditions — increased blood pressure, a high blood sugar level, excess body fat around the waist and abnormal cholesterol levels — that occur together, increasing your risk of heart disease, stroke and diabetes.

Metabolism: the process by which your body converts what you consume into energy

Monounsaturated and Polyunsaturated Fat: these fats protect against cardiovascular disease by promoting healthier serum lipid profiles: reducing LDL cholesterol and increasing HDL cholesterol.

Non-Alcoholic Fatty Liver Disease (NAFLD): when fat is deposited in the liver due to causes other than excessive alcohol consumption; it is related to insulin resistance and metabolic syndrome

Obesity: classified as having a BMI of 30.0 or over

Overweight: classified as having a BMI between 25.0 and 29.9

Serotonin: a neurotransmitter derived from the essential amino acid tryptophan; it contributes to the regulation of mood, appetite, and sleep

Sucrose: a compound that is the chief component of cane or beet sugar; pure white refined sugar

Telomeres: an essential part of cells that affects how long they can age; a sequence of DNA at the end of chromosomes

Toxin: a substance capable of causing injury or death; poisonous

Trans Fat: a type of fat produced industrially from vegetable fats for use in snack food, baked goods, and fast foods; consumption of trans fats increases the risk of cardiovascular disease by raising levels of LDL and lowering levels of HDL

Triglycerides: high levels of this blood lipid are associated with athero-sclerosis and heart disease

Tryptophan: an essential amino acid in the human diet that is a precursor of serotonin and may therefore improve depression symptoms

Type 1 Diabetes: a chronic condition, usually in childhood, where the pancreas produces little or no insulin resulting in hyperglycemia

Type 2 Diabetes: a chronic condition, usually in adults but becoming more common in children, characterized by hyperglycemia in the context of insulin resistance and relative lack of insulin

Ventral Tegmental Area (VTA): a part of the brain that releases dopamine

Ventromedial Hypothalamus (VMH): controls energy storage vs. expenditure

Very Low-Density Lipoproteins (VLDL): even bigger, bulkier, and more cumbersome than the "bad cholesterol" LDLs from trans fats; these clusters are prone to causing traffic jams in the bloodstream and arteries

Notes

Chapter 1:

1 Mark Aronson and Marina Budhos, *Sugar Changed the World: A Story of Magic, Spice, Slavery, Freedom, and Science* (New York: Clarion Books, 2010).

2 Lallanji Gopal, "Sugar-Making in Ancient India," *Journal of the Economic and Social History of the Orient* vol. 7, no. 1 (1964): 57-72.

3 Quoted in Mary Boyce, "Iranian Festivals," *The Cambridge History of Iran*, vol. 3(2), ed. E. Yarshater (Cambridge: Cambridge University Press, 1983), 798.

4 Virginia Mescher, *"How Sweet It Is!": A History of Sugar and Sugar Refining in the United States*, 2005.

5 Kate Hopkins, *Sweet Tooth: The Bittersweet History of Candy* (New York: St. Martin's Press, 2012).

6 Mark Aronson and Marina Budhos, *Sugar Changed the World: A Story of Magic, Spice, Slavery, Freedom, and Science* (New York: Clarion Books, 2010).

7 David Eltis, "The Slave Economies of the Caribbean: Structure, Performance, Evolution and Significance," *General History of the Caribbean* vol. 3, ed. Franklin W. Wright (London: UNESCO Publishing, 1997): 105-137.

Chapter2:

8 Voltaire, *Candide and Other Stories*, trans. Tobias Smollett (Digireads, 2009):36-37.

9 Edwin J. Perkins, *The Economy of Colonial America*, 2nd ed. (New York: Columbia University Press, 1988).

10 Quoted in K. Dian Kriz, "Sugar and the Specter of Cannibalism," *Sugar and the Visual Imagination in the Atlantic World* (Brown University, 2013).

11 Harvey Levenstein, *Revolution at the Table: The Transformation of the American Diet* (New York: Oxford University Press, 1988).

12 C.L.R. James, quoted in Jim Thomson, "The Haitian Revolution and the Forging of America," *The History Teacher* vol. 34, no. 1 (2000): 76-94.

13 Charley Richard, "200 Years of Progress in the Louisiana Sugar Industry: A Brief History," *American Sugar Cane League*.

14 Sidney W. Mintz, *Sweetness and Power: The Place of Sugar in Modern History* (New York: Penguin Books, 1985).

15 H.C. Prinsen Geerligs, *The World's Cane Sugar Industry* (Cambridge: Cambridge University Press, 1912).

16 Cathy K. Kaufman, "Salvation in Sweetness? Sugar Beets in Antebellum America," *Vegetables: Proceedings from the Oxford Symposium on Food and Cookery 2008*, Susan R. Friedland, ed. (Blackawton: Prospect Books, 2008): 95-104.

Chapter3:

17 Rakesh Chandra Tyagi, *Problems and Prospects of Sugar Industry in India* (New Delhi: Mittal Publications, 1995).

18 Mark Aronson and Marina Budhos, *Sugar Changed the World: A Story of Magic, Spice, Slavery, Freedom, and Science* (New York: Clarion Books, 2010).

19 Mark Twain, "The High Chief of Sugardom," The Sacramento *Daily Union*, 26 September 1866.

20 *Hawaiian Islands. Report of the Committee on Foreign Relations, United States Senate, with accompanying testimony, and Executive documents transmitted to Congress from January 1, 1883 to March 10, 1894*, page 1253.

21 D.H. Figueredo and Frank Argote-Freyre, *A Brief History of the Caribbean* (New York: Infobase Publishing, 2008).

22 Elizabeth Abbott, *Sugar: A Bittersweet History* (New York: Overlook Press, 2008).

23 Susan Salisbury, "Florida Crystals' 50th Anniversary a Landmark in Family's Journey," Palm Beach *Post* (October 28, 2010).

24 Jared Diamond, *Guns, Germs, and Steel: The Fates of Human Societies* (New York: W.W. Norton & Co., 1997).

25 Sucden, "World Sugar Trade." 2014. http://www.sucden.com/statistics/13_world-sugar-trade.

26 The United States Department of Labor, Bureau of International Labor Affairs, "List of Goods Produced by Child or Forced Labor," http://www.dol.gov/ilab/reports/child-labor/list-of-goods/.

27 Tom Phillips, "Brazilian Taskforce Frees More than 4,500 Slaves After Record Number of Raids on Remote Farms," *The Guardian* (January 2, 2009).

28 Simon Romero, "Spoonfuls of Hope, Tons of Pain; In Brazil's Sugar Empire, Workers Struggle with Mechanization," New York *Times* (May 21, 2000).

29 CSCC, *Dominican Sugar: A Macro View of Today's Industry*, 2011. http://assets.coca-colacompany.com/e5/1a/cd3d5c2b49ab93599bbb8200716d/DominicanSugarIndustry-AMacroLevelReport.pdf.

Chapter 4:

30 Richard Thomas Williamson, *Diabetes Mellitus and its Treatment* (New York: The Macmillan Company, 1898), 378-379.

31 Gary Taubes, *Good Calories, Bad Calories: Fats, Carbs, and the Controversial Science of Diet and Heatlh* (New York: First Anchor Books, 2008).

32 John Davis Billings, *Hard Tack and Coffee: or, the Unwritten Story of Army Life* (Boston: George W. Smith & Co., 1888), 130.

33 Ibid., 124.

34 Harvey Levenstein, *Revolution at the Table: The Transformation of the American Diet* (New York: Oxford University Press, 1988).

35 Ibid.

36 Freeman J. Bumstead and Robert W. Taylor, quoted in

37 Mark Pendergrast, *For God, Country, & Coca-Cola* (New York: Basic Books, 2013).

38 Quoted in Ibid.

39 John Harvey Kellogg, *Plain Facts for Old and Young* (Burlington: Segner & Condit, 1881), 183.

40 "An Evil which Needs to be Suppressed," *Modern Medicine and Bacteriological Review* vol. 5, no. 8 (1898): 194-195.

41 Ibid.

42 Harvey Levenstein, *Revolution at the Table: The Transformation of the American Diet* (New York: Oxford University Press, 1988).

43 Quoted in Martha M. Allen, "The W.C.T.U. and Coca Cola," *The Druggists Circular,* vol. 51 (December 1907), 784.

44 Quoted in Clayton A. Coppin and Jack High, *The Politics of Purity: Harvey Washington Wiley and the Origins of Federal Food Policy* (Ann Arbor: University of Michigan, 1999), 151.

45 Ludy T. Benjamin, "Pop Psychology: The Man Who Saved Coca-Cola," *Monitor on Psychology* 40, no. 2 (2009): 18.

46 "General News Items," *The Pennsylvania Medical Journal* vol. 15 (1912): 581.

47 Michael Pollan, "The (Agri)Cultural Contradictions of Obesity," New York *Times* (October 12, 2003).

Chapter 5:

48 Washington State University, "Annual Income Spent on Food," *Washington State Magazine* http://wsm.wsu.edu/researcher/2011fall_hunger_foodcost.php.

49 Michael Pollan, "What's Eating America," *Smithsonian* Magazine (July 2006).

50 The Sugar Association, "Why We Filed," http://sugar.org/cra-lawsuit/why-we-filed/.

51 John S. White, "Straight Talk about High-Fructose Corn Syrup: What it is and What it Ain't," *American Journal of Clinical Nutrition* vol. 88S (2008): 1716S-1721S.

52 Corn Refiners Association, "Educational Outreach," http://sweetsurprise.com/hfcs-educational-outreach.

53 Geraldine A. June to Audrae Erickson, July 3, 2008. http://www.corn.org/wp-content/uploads/2008/07/FDAdecision7-7-08.pdf.

54 Corn Refiners Association, "Corn Refiners Counter Sue the Sugar Association for Deceiving Consumers about High Fructose Corn Syrup" (September 4, 2012). http://www.corn.org/press/newsroom/corn-refiners-counter-sue-sugar-association/.

55 Quoted in Tom Hamburger, "'Soft Lobbying' War between Sugar, Corn Syrup Shows New Tactics in Washington Influence," Washington *Post* (February 12, 2014).

56 Corn Refiners Association, "Corn Refiners Counter Sue the Sugar Association for Deceiving Consumers about High Fructose Corn Syrup" (September 4, 2012). http://www.corn.org/press/newsroom/corn-refiners-counter-sue-sugar-association/.

57 Tom Hamburger, "'Soft Lobbying' War between Sugar, Corn Syrup Shows New Tactics in Washington Influence," Washington *Post* (February 12, 2014).

58 Quoted in Gary Taubes and Cristin Kearns Couzens, "Big Sugar's Sweet Little Lies," *Mother Jones* (November/December 2012).

59 Sugar Information, Inc., Advertisement, *LIFE* (November 13, 1970).

60 Sugar Information, Inc., Advertisement, *LIFE* (June 25, 1965).

61 Quoted in Gary Taubes and Cristin Kearns Couzens, "Big Sugar's Sweet Little Lies," *Mother Jones* (November/December 2012).

62 Marion Nestle, *Food Politics: How the Food Industry Influences Nutrition and Health* (Berkeley: University of California Press, 2002).

63 Barry M. Popkin and S.J. Nielsen, "The Sweetening of the World's Diet," *Obesity Research* vol. 11, no. 11 (2003): 1325-1332.

64 The Coca-Cola Company, "The Chronicle of Coca-Cola: A Symbol of Friendship," http://www.coca-colacompany.com/history.

65 USDA Economic Research Service, http://www.ers.usda.gov.

66 The Coca-Cola Company, "Per Capita Consumption of Company Beverage Products" (2012). http://www.coca-colacompany.com/annual-review/2012/pdf/2012-per-capita-consumption.pdf.

67 Derek Thompson, "How America Spends Money: 100 Years in the Life of the Family Budget," *The Atlantic* (April 5, 2012).

Chapter 6:

68 Domino Sugar. Advertisement, *LIFE* (September 28, 1953): 67.

69 Quoted in Laura T. Coffey, "Study: Some Cereals More than 50% Sugar," *Today* (October 2, 2009).

70 Harvey Levenstein, *Fear of Food: A History of Why We Worry about What We Eat* (Chicago: The University of Chicago Press, 2012).

Chapter 8:

71 Lennie, Terry, "The Metabolic Syndrome," *Circulation* vol. 114 (2006): e528-e529.

72 Andrew A. Bremer, et. al, "Toward a Unifying Hypothesis of Metabolic Syndrome," *Pediatrics* vol. 129, no. 3 (2012): 557-570.

73 Paul A. Heidenreich, et. al, "Forecasting the Future of Cardiovascular Disease in the United States: A Policy Statement from the American Heart Association," *Circulation* vol. 123 (2011): 933-944.

74 "Improvement of Gastroesophageal Reflux Disease After Initiation of a Low-Carbohydrate Diet: Five Brief Case Reports." W. S. Yancy, Jr, D. Provenzale, E. C. Westman Altern Ther Health Med. 2001 Nov-Dec; 7(6): 120, 116-9.

75 "A Very Low-Carbohydrate Diet Improves Gastroesophageal Reflux And Its Symptoms."Gregory L. Austin, Michelle T. Thiny, Eric C. Westman, William S. Yancy, Jr, Nicholas J. Shaheen Dig Dis Sci. 2006 August.

Chapter 9:

76 Centers for Disease Control and Prevention. National Diabetes Fact Sheet: National Estimates and General Information on Diabetes and Prediabetes in the United States, 2011.

77 James P. Boyle, et. al, "Projection of Diabetes Burden Through 2050: Impact of Changing Demography and Disease Prevalence in the U.S." *Diabetes Care* vol. 24, no. 11 (2001).

78 Matthias B. Schulze, et. al. "Sugar-Sweetened Beverages, Weight Gain, and Incidence of Type 2 Diabetes in Yound and Middle-Aged Women," *Journal of the American Medical Association*, vol. 292, no. 8 (2004): 927-934.

79 Laura Gabriela Sánchez-Lozada, et. al, "How Safe is Fructose for Persons With or Without Diabetes?" *American Journal of Clinical Nutrition* vol. 88, no. 5 (2008): 1189-1190.

80 International Diabetes Foundation, *IDF Diabetes Atlas, 6ᵗʰ edn.* (Brussels, Belgium: International Diabetes Foundation, 2013). http://www.idf.org/diabetesatlas.

81 American Diabetes Association, *Economic Costs of Diabetes in the U.S. in 2012.* http://www.diabetes.org.

Chapter 10:

82 Ali H. Mokdad, et. al, "The Spread of the Obesity Epidemic in the United States, 1991-1998." *Journal of the American Medical Association* vol. 282, no. 16 (1999): 1519-1522.

83 Aviva Must, et. al, "The Disease Burden Associated with Overweight and Obesity," *Journal of the American Medical Association* vol. 282, no. 16 (1999): 1523-1529.

84 Centers for Disease Control and Prevention, "Consumption of Added Sugar Among U.S. Children and Adolescents, 2005-2008." *NCHS Data Brief* no. 87 (2012).

85 Marion Nestle, *Food Politics: How the Food Industry Influences Nutrition and Health* (Berkeley: University of California Press, 2002).

86 Robert H. Lustig, *Fat Chance: Beating the Odds Against Sugar, Processed Food, Obesity, and Disease* (New York: Penguin Group, 2012).

87 Vecker, Todd. "Change Your Receptors, Change Your Set Point." *Getting Stronger.* N.p., 25 Oct. 2010. Web. 07 Aug. 2015.

88 William Nseir, et. al, "Soft Drinks Consumption and Nonalcoholic Fatty Liver Disease," *World Journal of Gastroenterology* vol. 16, no. 21 (2010): 2579-2588.

89 Ibid.

90 Robert H. Lustig, *Fat Chance: Beating the Odds Against Sugar, Processed Food, Obesity, and Disease* (New York: Penguin Group, 2012).

91 Sharon Begley, "As America's Waistline Expands, Costs Soar," *Reuters* April 30, 2012.

92 Donna M. Gates, et. al, "Obesity and Presenteeism: The Impact of Body Mass Index on Workplace Productivity," *Journal of Occupational & Environmental Science* vol. 50, no. 1 (2008): 39-45.

Chapter 11:

93 John P. Bantle, et. al, "Effects of Dietary Fructose on Plasma Lipids in Healthy Subjects," *American Journal of Clinical Nutrition* vol. 72, no. 5 (2000): 1128-1134.

94 Jean A. Welsh, et. al, "Caloric Sweetener Consumption and Dyslipidemia among US Adults," *Journal of the American Medical Association* vol. 303, no. 15 (2010): 1490-1497.

95 C.G. Beebe, et. al, "Blood Pressure of Rats as Affected by Diet and Concentration of NaCl in Drinking Water," *Proceedings of the Society for Experimental Biology and Medicine* vol. 151, no. 2 (1976): 395-399.

96 Richard A. Ahrens, et. al, "Moderate Sucrose Ingestion and Blood Pressure in the Rat," *Journal of Nutrition* vol. 110, no. 4 (1980): 725-731.

97 Wolfgang C. Winkelmayer, "Habitual Caffeine Intake and the Risk of Hypertension in Women," *Journal of the American Medical Association* vol. 294, no. 18 (2005): 2330-2335.

98 Paul A. Heidenreich, et. al, "Forecasting the Future of Cardiovascular Disease in the United States: A Policy Statement from the American Heart Association," *Circulation* vol. 123 (2011): 933-944.

Chapter 12:

99 Lois Baker, "Study Shows Glucose Consumption Increases Production of Destructive Free Radicals, Lowers Level of Key Antioxidant," State University of New York at Buffalo *News Center* (August 16, 2000).

100 Nobuyuki Sasaki, et. al, "Advanced Glycation End Products in Alzheimer's Disease and Other Neurodegenerative Diseases," *American Journal of Pathology* vol. 153, no. 4 (1998): 1149-1155.

101 Alzheimer's Association, "2013 Alzheimer's Disease Facts and Figures," *Alzheimer's & Dementia* vol. 9, no. 2 (2013).

102 Alison Goldin, et. al, "Advanced Glycation End Products: Sparking the Development of Diabetic Vascular Injury," *Circulation* vol. 114 (2006): 597-605.

103 Martha Clare Morris, et. al, "Dietary Intake of Antioxidant Nutrients and the Risk of Incident Alzheimer Disease in a Biracial Community Study," *Journal of the American Medical Association* vol. 287, no. 24 (2002): 3230-3237.

104 Li Jiao, et. al, "Advanced Glycation End Products, Soluble Receptor for Advanced Glycation End Products, and Risk of Colorectal Cancer," *Cancer Epidemiology, Biomarkers & Prevention* vol. 20, no. 7 (2011): 1430.

105 K.A. Moy, et. al, "Soluble Receptor for Advanced Glycation End Products and Risk of Liver Cancer," *Hepatology* vol. 57, no. 6 (2013): 2338-2345.

106 American Cancer Society, "Cancer Facts and Figures," (2014).

107 Natasa Tasevska, et. al, "Sugars in Diet and Risk of Cancer in the NIH-AARP Diet and Health Study," *International Journal of Cancer* vol. 130, no. 1 (2012): 159-169.

108 Isabelle Romieu, et. al, "Carbohydrates and the Risk of Breast Cancer Among Mexican Women," *Cancer Epidemiology, Biomarkers & Prevention* vol. 13 (2004): 1283-1289.

109 Dominique S. Michaud, et. al, "Dietary Glycemic Load, Carbohydrate, Sugar, and Colorectal Cancer Risk in Men and Women," *Cancer Epidemiology, Biomarkers & Prevention* vol. 14, no. 1 (2005): 138-143.

110 Emilie Friberg, et. al, "Sucrose, High-Sugar Foods, and Risk of Endometrial Cancer: A Population-Based Cohort Study," *Cancer Epidemiology, Biomarkers & Prevention* vol. 20 (2011): 1831-1837.

111 Gary Taubes, *Good Calories, Bad Calories: Challenging the Conventional Wisdom on Diet, Weight Control, and Disease* (New York: Alfred A. Knopf, 2007).

112 American Cancer Society, "Facts and Figures" (2014).

Chapter 13:

113 Quoted in Marc Aronson and Marina Budhos, *Sugar Changed the World: A Story of Magic, Spice, Slavery, Freedom, and Science* (New York: Clarion Books, 2010), 23.

114 Centers for Disease Control and Prevention, "Hygiene-Related Diseases: Dental Caries (Tooth Decay)," http://www.cdc.gov/healthywater/hygiene/disease/dental_caries.html.

115 Quoted in David N. Durant, *Where Queen Elizabeth Slept and What the Butler Saw* (New York: St. Martin's Press, 1996), 101.

116 John Yudkin, *Pure, White and Deadly* (London: Penguin, 1972).

117 L.M. Sreebny, "Sugar Availability, Sugar Consumption and Dental Caries," *Community Dentistry and Oral Epidemiology* vol. 10, no. 1 (1982): 1-7.

118 Riva Touger-Decker and Cor van Loveren, "Sugars and Dental Caries," *American Journal of Clinical Nutrition* vol. 78, no. 4 (2003): 881S-892S.

119 Ibid.

120 W. Sohn, et. al, "Carbonated Soft Drinks and Dental Caries in the Primary Dentition," *Journal of Dental Research* vol. 85, no. 3 (2006): 262-266.

121 K.E. Heller, et. al, "Sugared Soda Consumption and Dental Caries in the United States," *Journal of Dental Research* vol. 80, no. 10 (2001): 1949-1953.

122 Riva Touger-Decker and Cor van Loveren, "Sugars and Dental Caries," *American Journal of Clinical Nutrition* vol. 78, no. 4 (2003): 881S-892S.

123 W.J. Moore and E. Corbett, "The Distribution of Dental Caries in Ancient British Populations," *Caries Research* vol. 7, no. 2 (1973): 139-153.

124 Centers for Disease Control, "Achievements in Public Health, 1900-1999: Fluoridation of Drinking Water to Prevent Dental Caries," *Morbidity and Mortality Weekly Report* vol. 48, no. 41 (1999): 933-940.

125 Centers for Disease Control and Prevention, "Ten Great Public Health Achievements in the 20th Century," http://www.cdc.gov/about/history/tengpha.htm.

126 Riva Touger-Decker and Cor van Loveren, "Sugars and Dental Caries," *American Journal of Clinical Nutrition* vol. 78, no. 4 (2003): 881S-892S.

127 New York State Department of Health, "Fluoridation in New York State: Costs and Savings" (2014). https://www.health.ny.gov/prevention/dental/fluoridation/cost.htm.

Chapter 14:

128 Julie A. Mennella, et. al, "Preferences for Salty and Sweet Tastes are Elevated and Related to Each Other During Childhood," *PLoS ONE* vol. 9, no. 3 (2014): e92201.

129 Nancy F. Butte, "The Role of Breastfeeding in Obesity," *Pediatric Clinics of North America* vol. 48, no. 1 (2001): 189-198.

130 Adam Drewnowski, et. al, "Sweetness and Food Preference," *Journal of Nutrition* vol. 142, no. 6 (2012): 1142S-1148S.

131 Charlene D. Elliott, "Sweet and Salty: Nutritional Content and Analysis of Baby and Toddler Foods," *Journal of Public Health* (2010) doi: 10.1093/pubmed/fdq037.

132 Sloveig A. Cunningham, et. al, "Incidence of Childhood Obesity in the United States," *New England Journal of Medicine* vol. 370, no. 5 (2014): 403-411.

Chapter 15:

133 O. Arrias-Carrión and E. Pöppel, "Dopamine, Learning and Reward-Seeking Behavior," *Acta Neurobiologiae Experimentalis* vol. 67, no. 4 (2007): 481-488.

134 Volkow, Nora D., and Roy A. Wise. "How Can Drug Addiction Help Us Understand Obesity?" *Nature Neuroscience Nat Neurosci* 8.5 (2005): 555-60. Web.

135 Pedro Rada, et. al, "Daily Bingeing on Sugar Repeatedly Releases Dopamine in the Accumbens Shell," *Neuroscience* vol. 134, no. 3 (2005): 737-744.

136 David A. Kessler, *The End of Overeating: Taking Control of the Insatiable American Appetite* (New York: Rodale, 2009).

137 Locker, Melissa. "Oreos May Be As Addictive As Cocaine," *TIME* (October 16, 2013).

138 J.R. Ifland, et. al, "Refined Food Addiction: A Classic Substance Use Disorder," *Medical Hypotheses* vol. 72, no. 5 (2009): 518-526.

139 N.A. Schvey, et. al, "The Stress of Stigma: Exploring the Effect of Weight Stigma on Cortisol Reactivity," *Psychosomatic Medicine* (2014): 1-7.

140 Kelli E. Friedman, et. al, "Recent Experiences of Weight-Based Stigmatization in a Weight Loss Surgery Population: Psychological and Behavioral Correlates," *Obesity* vol. 16, no. S2 (2008): S69-S74.

Chapter 16:

141 Donald T. Fullerton, et. al, "Sugar, Opioids, and Binge Eating," *Brain Research Bulletin* vol. 14, no. 6 (1985): 673-680.
142 Elliott M. Blass, "Phylogenetic and Ontogenetic Contributions to Today's Obesity Quagmire," *Food and Addiction* ed. Kelly D. Brownell and Mark S. Gold (Oxford: Oxford University Press, 2012): 172-177.
143 Elliott Blass, et. al, "Interactions Between Sucrose, Pain and Isolation Distress," *Pharmacology, Biochemistry & Behavior* vol. 26, no. 3 (1986): 483-489.
144 Ibid.
145 L. Christensen, "The Effect of Food Intake on Mood," *Clinical Nutrition* vol. 20, s. 1 (2001): 161-166.
146 Donald T. Fullerton, et. al, "Sugar, Opioids, and Binge Eating," *Brain Research Bulletin* vol. 14, no. 6 (1985): 673-680.
147 Rudolph Spangler, et. al, "Opiate-Like Effects of Sugar on Gene Expression in Reward Areas of the Rat Brain," *Molecular Brain Research* vol. 124, no. 2 (2004): 134-142.
148 Nicole M. Avena, et. al, "Evidence for Sugar Addiction: Behavioral and Neurochemical Effects of Intermittent, Excessive Sugar Intake," *Neuroscience & Biobehavioral Reviews* vol. 32, no. 1 (2008): 20-39.
149 Jim Gormally, et. al, "The Assessment of Binge Eating Severity Among Obese Persons," *Addictive Behaviors* vol. 7, no. 1 (1982): 47-55.

Chapter 17:

150 Robert C. Andrews and Brian R. Walker, "Glucocorticoids and Insulin Resistance: Old Hormones, New Targets," *Clinical Science* vol. 96 (1999): 513-523.
151 Susan J. Torres and Caryl A. Nowson, "Relationship Between Stress, Eating Behavior, and Obesity," *Nutrition* vol. 23, nos. 11-12 (2007): 887-894.
152 American Psychological Association, "Stress in America: Our Health at Risk," (2012).
153 Georgina Oliver and Jane Wardle, "Perceived Effects of Stress on Food Choice," *Physiology & Behavior* vol. 66, no. 3 (1999): 511-515.
154 American Psychological Association, "Stress in America: Our Health at Risk," (2012).

Chapter 18:

155 Thomas Insel, "Antidepressants: A Complicated Picture," National Institute for Mental Health (2011).
156 Simon N. Young, "How to Increase Serotonin in the Human Brain without Drugs," *Journal of Psychiatry & Neuroscience* vol. 32, no. 6 (2007): 394-399.
157 Michael Voracek and Ulrich S. Tran, "Dietary Tryptophan Intake and Suicide Rate in Industrialized Nations," *Journal of Affective Disorders* vol. 98, no. 3 (2007): 259-262.

158 Arthur N. Westover and Lauren B. Marangell, "A Cross-National Relationship Between Sugar Consumption and Major Depression?" *Depression and Anxiety* vol. 16, no. 3 (2002): 118-120.

159 Chrystal Moulton, "Consumption of Alcohol Leads to a 26% Reduction in Plasma Tryptophan Levels," Natural Health Research Institute (2014).

Chapter 19:

160 Mike Esterl, "Forget Dinner. It's Always Snack Time in America," *Wall Street Journal* (July 2, 2014).

161 D.M. Gates, et. al, "Obesity and Presenteeism: The Impact of Body Mass Index on Workplace Productivity," *Journal of Occupational and Environmental Medicine* vol. 50, no. 1 (2008): 39-45.

162 E.A. Finkelstein, et. al, "The Costs of Obesity in the Workplace," *Journal of Occupational and Environmental Medicine* vol. 52, no. 10 (2010): 971-976.

163 American Psychiatric Association. *Diagnostic and Statistical Manual of Mental Disorders,* fifth edition (Arlington, VA: American Psychiatric Association, 2013).

164 Youfa Wang, et. al, "Will All Americans Become Overweight or Obese? Estimating the Progression and Cost of the US Obesity Epidemic," *Obesity* vol. 16, no. 10 (2008): 2323-2330.

Chapter 20:

165 Robert H. Lustig, *Fat Chance: Beating the Odds Against Sugar, Processed Food, Obesity, and Disease* (New York: Penguin Group, 2012).

166 Ashley N. Gearhardt, et. al, "Neural Correlates of Food Addiction," *Journal of the American Medical Association of Psychiatry* vol. 68, no. 8 (2011): 808-816.

167 Nicole M. Avena, et. al, "Evidence for Sugar Addiction: Behavioral and Neurochemical Effects of Intermittent, Excessive Sugar Intake," *Neuroscience & Biobehavioral Reviews* vol. 32, no. 1 (2008): 20-39.

168 Jeffrey L. Fortuna, "Sweet Preference, Sugar Addiction and the Familial History of Alcohol Dependence: Shared Neural Pathways and Genes," *Journal of Psychoactive Drugs* vol. 42, no. 2 (2010): 147-151.

169 A. Kampov-Polevoy, et. al, "Evidence of Preference for a High-Concentration Sucrose Solution in Alcoholic Men," *American Journal of Psychiatry* vol. 154, no. 2 (1997): 269-270.

170 Jeffrey L. Fortuna, "Sweet Preference, Sugar Addiction and the Familial History of Alcohol Dependence: Shared Neural Pathways and Genes," *Journal of Psychoactive Drugs* vol. 42, no. 2 (2010): 147-151.

171 Kathleen DesMaisons, *Potatoes Not Prozac* (New York: Simon & Schuster, 1998).

172 D.M. Dick and L.J. Beirut, "The Genetics of Alcohol Dependence," *Current Psychiatric Reports* vol. 8, no. 2 (2006): 151-157.

Chapter 21:

173 Mission: Readiness, Military Leaders for Kids, "Too Fat to Fight: Retired Military Leaders Want Junk Food Out of America's Schools," (2010).

174 Ross DeVol and Armen Bedroussian, *An Unhealthy America: The Economic Burden of Chronic Disease.* Milken Institute (October 2007).

Chapter 22:

175 Benjamin Caballero, et. al, "Pathways: A School-Based, Randomized Controlled Trial for the Prevention of Obesity in American Indian Schoolchildren," *American Journal of Clinical Nutrition* vol. 78, no. 5 (2003): 1030-1038.

176 Megan E. LaDolce, et. al, "Sugar as Part of a Balanced Breakfast? What Cereal Advertisements Teach Children about Healthy Eating." *Journal of Health Communication* (2013).

177 Centers for Disease Control and Prevention, "Basics About Childhood Obesity," (2014): http://www.cdc.gov/obesity/childhood/basics.html.

178 Laura T. Coffey, "Study: Some Cereals More than 50% Sugar," *Today* (October 2, 2009).

179 Institute of Medicine, *Food Marketing to Children and Youth: Threat or Opportunity?* (2005).

180 Quoted in J. Howard Beales, "Advertising to Kids and the FTC: A Regulatory Retrospective that Advises the Present" (Federal Trade Commission: 2004).

181 Quoted in William H. Dietz, "New Strategies to Improve Food Marketing to Children," *Health Affairs* vol. 32, no. 9 (2013): 1652-1658.

182 Quoted in Bridget Huber, "Michelle Obama's Moves." *The Nation* October 29, 2012. http://www.thenation.com/article/170485/michelles-moves#.

183 Centers for Disease Control and Prevention, www.cdc.gov.

184 "The Real Bears," directed by Lucas Zanotto (2012; Boulder, CO and Austin, TX: Common and the Butler Brothers). http://www.therealbears.org/.

185 Quoted in Mark Bittman, "Food's Big-Picture Guy," New York *Times* (May 27, 2014)

Chapter 23:

186 Food Research and Action Center, "Relationship Between Hunger and Overweight or Obesity," http://frac.org/initiatives/hunger-and-obesity/are-hunger-and-obesity-related/.

187 E.B. Loucks, et. al, "Socioeconomic Disparities in Metabolic Syndrome Differ by Gender: Evidence from NHANES III," *Annals of Epidemiology* vol. 17, no. 1 (2007): 19-26.

188 James A. Levine, "Poverty and Obesity in the U.S.," *Diabetes* vol. 60, no. 11 (2011): 2667-2668.

189 Barry M. Popkin, "The World is Fat," *Scientific American* (September 2007).

190 Jennifer Jabs and Carol M. Devine, "Time Scarcity and Food Choices: An Overview," *Appetite* vol. 47, no. 2 (2006): 196-204.

191 Tatiana Andreyeva, et. al, "Grocery Store Beverage Choices by Participants in Federal Food Assistance and Nutrition Programs," *American Journal of Preventative Medicine* vol. 43, no. 4 (2012): 411-418.

192 Stan Cox, "Big Soda SNAP-ing Up Billions off Government Programs," *Salon* (May 20, 2013).

193 Cindy W. Leung, et. al, "Associations of Food Stamp Participation with Dietary Quality and Obesity in Children," *Pediatrics* vol. 131, no. 3 (2013): 463-472.

194 Tatiana Andreyeva and Joerg Luedicke, "Incentivizing Fruit and Vegetable Purchases Among Participants in the Special Supplemental Nutrition Program for Women, Infants, and Children," *Public Health Nutrition* (2014): 1-9. doi: 10.1017/S1368980014000512.

195 Mayuree Rao, et. al, "Do Healthier Foods and Diet Patterns Cost More than Less Healthy Options? A Systematic Review and Meta-Analysis," *BMJ Open* vol. 3, no. 12 (2013): doi:10.1136/bmjopen-2013-004277.

196 Antronette K. Yancey, et. al, "A Cross-Sectional Prevalence Study of Ethnically Targeted and General Audience Outdoor Obesity-Related Advertising," *Milbank Quarterly* vol. 87, no. 1 (2009): 155-184.

197 Yale Rudd Center for Food Policy & Obesity, "Sugar Drink Targeted Marketing," (2011). http://sugarydrinkfacts.org.

Chapter 24:

198 Lisa L. Sharma, Stephen P. Teret, and Kelly D. Brownell, "The Food Industry and Self-Regulation: Standards to Promote Success and to Avoid Public Health Failures," *American Journal of Public Health* vol. 100, no. 2 (2010): 240-246.

199 FDA, "Draft Guidance for Industry: Ingredients Declared as Evaporated Cane Juice," http://www.fda.gov/food/guidanceregulation/guidancedocumentsre gulatoryinformation/labelingnutrition/ucm181491.htm

200 Christina A. Roberto, et. al, "Influence of Licensed Characters on Children's Taste and Snack Preferences," *Pediatrics* (2010) doi:10.1542/peds.2009-3433.

Chapter 25:

201 United States Department of Agriculture and United States Department of Health and Human Services, *2010 Dietary Guidelines for Americans* (2010).

202 American Heart Association, "Added Sugars," http://www.heart.org/HEARTORG/GettingHealthy/NutritionCenter/HealthyEati ng/Added-Sugars_UCM_305858_Article.jsp

203 Qing Yang, "Gain Weight by 'Going Diet?': Artificial Sweeteners and the Neurobiology of Sugar Cravings," *Yale Journal of Biology and Medicine* vol. 83, no. 2 (2010): 101-108.